Health Informatics
(formerly Computers in Health Care)

Kathryn J. Hannah   Marion J. Ball
Series Editors

Springer
New York
Berlin
Heidelberg
Barcelona
Budapest
Hong Kong
London
Milan
Paris
Singapore
Tokyo

Health Informatics
(formerly Computers in Health Care)

Series Editors:
Kathryn J. Hannah   Marion J. Ball

Dental Informatics
Integrating Technology into the Dental Environment
L.M. Abbey and J. Zimmerman

Aspects of the Computer-based Patient Record
M.J. Ball and M.F. Collen

Nursing Informatics
Where Caring and Technology Meet, Second Edition
M.J. Ball, K.J. Hannah, S.K. Newbold, and J.V. Douglas

Healthcare Information Management Systems
A Practical Guide, Second Edition
M.J. Ball, D.W. Simborg, J.W. Albright, and J.V. Douglas

Clinical Decision Support Systems
Theory and Practice
E.S. Berner

Strategy and Architecture of Health Care Information Systems
M.K. Bourke

Information Networks for Community Health
P.F. Brennan, S.J. Schneider, and E. Tornquist

Introduction to Medical Informatics
P. Degoulet and M. Fieschi

Patient Care Information Systems
Successful Design and Implementation
E.L. Drazen, J.B. Metzger, J.L. Ritter, and M.K. Schneider

Introduction to Nursing Informatics
K.J. Hannah, M.J. Ball, and M.J.A. Edwards

Computerizing Large Integrated Health Networks
The VA Success
R.M. Kolodner

Organizational Aspects of Health Informatics
Managing Technological Change
N.M. Lorenzi and R.T. Riley

Transforming Health Care Through Information
Case Studies
N.M. Lorenzi, R.T. Riley, M.J. Ball, and J.V. Douglas

(continued after Index)

Eta S. Berner
Editor

Clinical Decision Support Systems
Theory and Practice

With a Foreword by Marion J. Ball

With 11 Illustrations

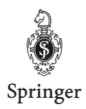

Springer

Eta S. Berner, EdD
Professor, Masters of Science in Health
Informatics Program
Department of Health Services
    Administration
School of Health Related Professions
and

Section of Medical Informatics
Division of General Medicine
Department of Medicine
School of Medicine
University of Alabama
1675 University Boulevard, Room 544
Birmingham, AL 35294-8219, USA

Series Editors:

Kathryn J. Hannah, PhD, RN
Leader, Health Informatics Group
Sierra Systems Consultants, Inc.
and
Professor, Department of Community
    Health Science
Faculty of Medicine
The University of Calgary
Calgary, Alberta, Canada

Marion J. Ball, EdD
Professor, Department of
    Epidemiology
University of Maryland School of
    Medicine
and
Vice President
First Consulting Group
Baltimore, MD, USA

Library of Congress Cataloging-in-Publication Data
Clinical decision support systems in theory and practice / [edited by]
    Eta S. Berner.
        p.   cm.—(Health informatics)
    Includes bibliographical references and index.
    ISBN 0-387-98575-1 (hardcover: alk. paper)
    1. Diagnosis—Decision making—Data processing.   2. Clinical
medicine—Decision making—Data processing.   3. Expert systems
(Computer science)   I. Berner, Eta S., 1946–.   II. Series.
    [DNLM: 1. Decision Support Systems, Clinical.   2. Diagnosis,
Computer-Assisted.   3. Expert Systems.   WB 141 C6371 1998]
    RC78.7.D35C55   1998
    616.07'5'0285—dc21
    DNLM/DLC   98—21883

Production coordinated by A. Orrantia; manufacturing supervised by Joe Quatela.
Photocomposed by Michelle M. Stroveglia, Massapequa, NY.
Printed and bound by Edwards Brothers, Inc., Ann Arbor, MI.
Printed in the United States of America.

9 8 7 6 5 4 3 2 1

ISBN 0-387-98575-1 Springer-Verlag New York Berlin Heidelberg   SPIN 10682325

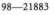

To David, Daniel, and Jacob

This exciting volume will illuminate our path as we enter the knowledge era of the 21st century. We find here real case studies that chronicle the successful use of decision support and expert systems in health care. In demonstrating the knowledge transfer process, these cases take what has been theory into the actual practice of medicine and health care delivery. These are changes of the highest order, and the transformation they promise is dependent upon our addressing two vital and very different components.

- One involves "peopleware" and requires that we bring cognitive scientists, behaviorists, and social scientists into health informatics.
- The other is highly technical and involves the "engine" that drives systems, creating knowledge and shaping health care delivery.

Both are essential components as we work to bring knowledge to where it is needed, be it the bedside, the home, the classroom, the office, or the research bench. Those of us who have labored to make health informatics a recognized discipline know the difficulties involved in taking new approaches to gathering data, seeking information, and creating knowledge. We need new tool sets and new mindsets as we enter the 21st century. This is a tall order, but it can be met, as this volume so richly demonstrates.

For added insights, we look to the work on organizational development reported by Nancy Lorenzi and Robert Riley earlier in the Computers in Health Care series. They address the "soft issues" that have proved to be hard realities in far too many information system implementations. We look to cognitive scientists, like Vimla Patel, who are showing us how we can make tools that are intuitive, responsive to and reflective of different learning and information-seeking styles.

The premise of this Springer series—and the conviction that has governed our professional lives—is that health informatics can improve care. Today the engine that drives health care information systems is more powerful than ever before. We are already realizing the benefit of new communication capabilities. And these promise to increase exponentially once advances like Sequoia's extended mark-up language (XML) solve the problems of data entry and file conversion, making health records shareable across the Internet, able to populate data warehouses and knowledge repositories.

As evidence-based medicine becomes a reality, we will be in for exciting times. Managing this knowledge-driven enterprise will require new skills, processes, and policies. But with these risks come new opportunities, for health care organizations and for individuals giving or receiving health care.

Preparing to enter this bold new world, we owe a tremendous debt of gratitude to Eta Berner and to the informaticians who contributed to this volume. Together they have given us the compass that will help guide us on our way.

Marion J. Ball

This series is directed to healthcare professionals who are leading the transformation of health care by using information and knowledge. Launched in 1988 as Computers in Health Care, the series offers a broad range of titles: some addressed to specific professions like nursing, medicine, or health administration; other to special areas of practice such as trauma or radiology. Still other books in the series focus on interdisciplinary issues like the computer-based patient record, electronic health records or networked healthcare systems.

Renamed Health Informatics in 1998, to reflect the rapid evolution in the discipline now known as health informatics, the series will continue to add titles that contribute to the continuing evolution of the field. In the series eminent experts, as editors or authors, offer their accounts of innovations in health informatics. Increasingly, these accounts go beyond hardware and software to address the role of information in influencing the transformation of health care delivery systems around the world. The series also will increasingly focus on "peopleware" and the organizational, behavioral and societal changes that accompany the diffusion of information technology in health services environments.

These changes will shape health services in the next millennium. By making full and creative use of the technology to tame data and to transform information, health informatics will foster the development of the knowledge age in health care. As co-editors, we pledge to support our professional colleagues and the series readers as they share advances in the emerging and exciting field of Health Informatics.

Kathryn J. Hannah
Marion J. Ball

PREFACE

We are at the beginning of a new era in the application of computer-based decision support for clinical medicine. The purpose of this book is to provide an overview of the state-of-the-art diagnostic computer applications, to identify the issues that will need to be addressed as these systems continue to evolve, and to serve as a comprehensive resource for physicians and other health professionals, medical and health informatics students, and researchers interested in the development and application of computer-based diagnostic tools.

This book is designed to be (1) a resource book on diagnostic systems for informatics specialists; (2) a textbook for teachers or students in health or medical informatics training programs; and (3) a comprehensive introduction for clinicians, with or without expertise in the applications of computers in medicine, who are interested in learning about current developments in computer-based diagnostic systems. In recent years, it has become obvious that other health professionals, in addition to physicians, have needs for decision support and that the issues raised in this book apply to this broad range of clinicians. The book includes chapters by nationally and internationally recognized experts on the design, evaluation and application of these systems who examine the impact of practitioner and patient use of computer-based diagnostic tools.

The field of health informatics, in its broadest definition, involves the development and use of systems for the management of health information. The computer-based systems that are described in this book focus on the management of information needed for patient diagnosis. The term "expert system" is often applied to computer-based systems that are expected to provide advice to clinicians. Although the label "expert system" has often been used loosely, virtually none of the systems in operation today function with the precision and degree of independence that would enable them to operate in isolation from the clinician-user, nor is it the intention of the developers of these systems that they do so. For one thing, these computer systems usually generate multiple diagnostic suggestions, rather than a single definitive diagnosis. Consequently, those who use the systems must arrive at a diagnosis by using their own knowledge and experience to review, process and adapt the information provided by the computer. G. Octo Barnett, M.D., one of the pioneers in the development of computer-based medical systems, has emphasized that the computer does not develop a differential diagnosis, the clinician does. Having appropriate expectations for the manner in which these systems function is essential to understanding the information contained in this book. For this reason we use the term "clinical diagnostic decision support system(s) (CDDSS)" for the tools that are described here. This terminology emphasizes that these systems are designed to provide information to assist and support the clinician with diagnostic decisions.

The book is divided into three sections, with several chapters in each section. Each chapter has extensive references for the reader who wishes to examine the individual research studies in detail.

Section I describes CDDSS development and performance evaluation. The first chapter provides an overview of the history of CDDSS and sets this development in the context of the process of physician, not just computer, diagnosis. In addition, chapter 1 outlines the major issues that are addressed in detail in the rest of the book. This chapter and the following chapter, which focuses on the mathematical foundations of diagnostic systems, provides the background needed to understand the other chapters. Chapter 3 summarizes the data on what is known to date on the evaluation of these systems.

Section II includes three chapters that describe a variety of applications of these systems. These applications include the use of CDDSS and other systems with diagnostic components linked to an online hospital information system (chapter 4), and applications of CDDSS in educational settings for medical students, residents, and allied health professionals (chapter 5). Chapter 6 describes a variety of computer-based applications that can be used by health care providers for patient education or by patients themselves, as part of their own search for medical and health information. Because there has been such an increase in medically related information sources for patients available online, we have included an Appendix with relevant addresses for Internet-based sites.

The last section deals with the issues that must be considered in wide-scale implementation. Chapter 7 discusses the design and implementation needs. Clinical trials of information interventions are addressed in chapter 8 and ethical concerns are discussed in chapter 9.

This book represents an effort, not just by the editor and the individual chapter authors, but by many others who have provided assistance to them. We wish to express our appreciation to the following individuals who reviewed and critiqued parts of this book: Herbert S. Waxman, M.D., for his review of chapter 3, Dr. William S. Yamamoto for his insightful comments on chapter 7, Professor Kathy L. Cerminara and other members of the University of Miami Health Law and Ethics Study Group for valuable comments on a draft of chapter 9, and Ms. Brook Watts for her review and feedback on the entire manuscript.

I would like to express my appreciation to Marion Ball and Kathryn Hannah, William Day and the production staff at Springer-Verlag who helped shepherd this book through the publication process. I would also like to recognize the efforts of Ms. Mary Sue B. Pruett, whose painstaking attention to detail in the preparation of this manuscript was invaluable. The National Library of Medicine, through grant RO1-LM 05125, has provided much appreciated support for my research on clinical diagnostic decision support systems. Finally, I want to express my gratitude to my colleague, C. Michael Brooks, Ed.D., without whose support and guidance, this book would not have been written.

Eta S. Berner
July 1998

CONTENTS

Foreword vii
Series Preface ix
Preface xi
Contributors xix

PART I
DEVELOPMENT AND EVALUATION OF
CLINICAL DIAGNOSTIC DECISION SUPPORT SYSTEMS

1. Clinical Diagnostic Decision Support Systems:
   An Overview 3
   Randolph A. Miller and Antoine Geissbuhler
   Definitions of Diagnosis 4
   Human Diagnostic Reasoning 9
   Historical Survey of CDDSS 13
   Developing, Implementing, Evaluating
      and Maintaining CDDSS 18
   Legal and Ethical Issues 28
   The Future of CDDSS 30

2. Mathematical Foundations of Decision Support Systems 35
   S. Andrew Spooner
   Review of Logic and Probability 36
   The General Model of Diagnostic Decision Support
      Systems 49
   Non-Knowledge-Based Systems 56
   Summary 58

3. Testing System Accuracy 61
   Eta S. Berner
   Performance of CDDSS 62
   Interpretation of Performance Data 65
   Conclusions 70

PART II
APPLICATIONS OF CLINICAL DIAGNOSTIC
DECISION SUPPORT SYSTEMS

4. Hospital-Based Decision Support 77
   Peter J. Haug, Reed M. Gardner and R. Scott Evans
   The HELP System 79
   Categories of Decision Support Technologies 80
   "Diagnostic" Decision Support with the HELP System 88
   Summary 99

5. Medical Education Applications 105
   Michael J. Lincoln
   Reasons to Adopt CDDSS in Medical Curricula 106
   The Nature of Medical CDDSS 108
   How CDDSS Can Enhance Clinical Problem Solving 111
   Examples of CDDSS in Medical Education 113
   Discussion 129
   Summary 133

6. Decision Support for Patients 139
   Holly Brügge Jimison and Paul Phillip Sher
   Role of Consumer Health Informatics in Patient Care 139
   The Computer as a Health Information Medium 141
   Diagnostic and Other Decision Support Systems
        for Patients 148
   Diagnostic Decision Support 153
   Patient Access to Diagnostic Decision Support Systems 159
   The Future of Diagnostic Decision Support Systems
        for Patients 162

PART III
FUTURE DEVELOPMENT OF
CLINICAL DIAGNOSTIC DECISION SUPPORT SYSTEMS

7. Design and Implementation Issues 169
   Jerome H. Carter
   Technical Design Issues 171
   Reasoning 178
   Knowledge Acquisition 187
   Human-Computer Interaction 191
   Systems Integration 193
   Conclusion 194

8. Clinical Trials of Information Interventions 199
   E. Andrew Balas and Suzanne Austin Boren
   The Practical and Scientific Need for Clinical Testing 200
   Research Methods of Demonstrating Practical Impact 201
   User Satisfaction with Decision Support Systems 203
   Randomized Controlled Clinical Trials of Decision
        Support Services 204
   Columbia Registry of Medical Management Trials 207

9. Ethical and Legal Issues in Decision Support 217
   Kenneth W. Goodman
   Ethical Issues 218
   Legal and Regulatory Issues 226
   Conclusion and Future Directions 231

Afterword 235

Appendix: Examples of Internet Resources for Patients 237

References 239

Index 261

CONTRIBUTORS

E. Andrew Balas, MD, PhD
Health Services Management,
University of Missouri,
Columbia, Missouri, USA

Suzanne Austin Boren, MHA
Health Services Management,
University of Missouri,
Columbia, Missouri, USA

Eta S. Berner, EdD
Master of Science in Health Informatics Program,
Department of Health Services Administration,
School of Health Related Professions,
and
Section of Medical Informatics,
Division of General Medicine,
Department of Medicine,
School of Medicine,
University of Alabama at Birmingham,
Birmingham, Alabama, USA

Jerome H. Carter, MD
Section of Medical Informatics,
Division of General Medicine,
Department of Medicine,
University of Alabama at Birmingham,
Birmingham, Alabama, USA

R. Scott Evans, PhD
Clinical Epidemiology,
LDS Hospital/University of Utah,
Salt Lake City, Utah, USA

Reed M. Gardner, PhD
Department of Medical Informatics,
LDS Hospital/University of Utah,
Salt Lake City, Utah, USA

Antoine Geissbuhler, MD
Division of Biomedical Informatics,
Vanderbilt University Medical Center,
Nashville, Tennessee, USA

Kenneth W. Goodman, PhD
Forum for Bioethics and Philosophy,
University of Miami,
Miami, Florida, USA

Peter J. Haug, MD
Department of Medical Informatics,
LDS Hospital/University of Utah,
Salt Lake City, Utah, USA

Holly Brügge Jimison, PhD
Informed Patient Decisions Group,
Oregon Health Sciences University,
Portland, Oregon, USA

Michael J. Lincoln, MD
Internal Medicine and Medical Informatics,
Department of Veterans Affairs,
Salt Lake City VA Medical Center,
University of Utah School of School of Medicine,
Department of Medical Informatics,
Salt Lake City, Utah, USA

Randolph A. Miller, MD
Division of Biomedical Informatics,
Vanderbilt University Medical Center,
Nashville, Tennessee, USA

Paul Phillip Sher, MD
Oregon Health Sciences University,
Portland, Oregon, USA

S. Andrew Spooner, MD
Division of General Pediatrics,
Department of Pediatrics,
University of Alabama at Birmingham,
Birmingham, Alabama, USA

Part I

Development and Evaluation of Clinical Diagnostic Decision Support Systems

====== CHAPTER 1 ======

Clinical Diagnostic Decision Support Systems—An Overview*

Randolph A. Miller and Antoine Geissbuhler

Since primeval times, mankind has attempted to explain natural phenomena using models. For the past four decades a new kind of modeler, the health care informatician, has developed and proliferated a new kind of model, the Clinical Diagnostic Decision Support System (CDDSS). Modeling historically was, and still remains, an inexact science. Ptolemy, in the 'Almagest', placed the earth at the center of the universe, and could still explain why the sun would rise in the east each morning. Newton's nonrelativistic formulation of the laws of mechanics work well for earth-bound engineering applications. Past and present CDDSS incorporate inexact models of the incompletely understood and exceptionally complex process of clinical diagnosis. Yet mankind, using imperfect models, has built machines that fly and has cured many diseases. Because CDDSS augment the natural capabilities of human diagnosticians, it is likely they will be employed productively.[1]

* Portions of this chapter have been taken verbatim, with permission of the American Medical Informatics Association (AMIA), which owns the copyrights, from: Miller RA. Medical Diagnostic Decision Support Systems—Past, Present, and Future: A Threaded Bibliography and Commentary. JAMIA 1994; 1:8-27, and from Miller RA. Evaluating Evaluations of Medical Diagnostic Systems, JAMIA 1996; 3:429-431.

This chapter presents a definition of clinical diagnosis and of CDDSS; a discussion of how humans accomplish diagnosis; a survey of previous attempts to develop computer-based clinical diagnostic tools; a discussion of the problems encountered in developing, implementing, evaluating, and maintaining clinical diagnostic decision support systems; and a brief discussion of the future of such systems. Some of these topics are treated in more depth in subsequent chapters of this book.

DEFINITIONS OF DIAGNOSIS

In order to understand the history of clinical diagnostic decision support systems and envision their future roles, it is important to define clinical diagnosis and computer-assisted clinical diagnosis. A simple definition of diagnosis is:[2]

> *the placing of an interpretive, higher level label on a set of raw, more primitive observations* [Definition 1].

By this definition one form of diagnosis might consist of labeling, as "abnormal", any laboratory test results falling outside 1.5 times the 95% confidence intervals for the "normal" values seen in the general population as measured by that laboratory. Another level of diagnosis under the same definition might consist of labeling the combination of a low serum bicarbonate level, a high serum chloride level, and an arterial blood pH of 7.3 as "metabolic acidosis".

A more involved definition of diagnosis, specific for clinical diagnosis, is:[2]

> *a mapping from a patient's data (normal and abnormal history, physical examination, and laboratory data) to a nosology of disease states* [Definition 2].

Both of these definitions treat diagnosis improperly as a single event, rather than as a process. A more accurate definition is found in the Random House Collegiate Dictionary. There diagnosis is defined as:[3]

> *"the process of determining by examination the nature and circumstances of a diseased condition"* [Definition 3].

Skilled diagnosticians develop an understanding of what the patient's life situation was like before the illness began, how the illness has manifested itself, and how it has affected the life situation.[2] The clinician must also determine the patient's understanding of, and response to, an illness. The process of diagnosis entails a sequence of interdependent, often highly individualized, tasks: evoking from the patient's initial history and physical examination findings; integration of the data into plausible scenarios regarding known disease processes; evaluating and refining diagnostic hypotheses through selective elicitation of additional patient information, such as laboratory tests or serial examinations; initiating therapy at appropriate points in time (including before a diagnosis is established); and evaluating the effect of both the illness and the therapy on the patient over time.[2]

Diagnosis is a process composed of individual steps. These steps go from a point of origin (a question and a set of "presenting findings" and "previously established diagnoses"), to a point of destination (an answer, usually consisting of a set of "new established diagnoses" and/or "unresolved differential diagnoses"). While the beginning and end points may be identical, the steps one diagnostician follows may be very different from those taken by another diagnostician, and the same diagnostician may take different steps in two nearly identical cases. Because expertise varies among clinicians, different individuals will encounter different diagnostic problems in evaluating the same patient. For instance, they may generate dissimilar questions based on difficulties with disparate steps in the diagnostic process, even if they follow exactly the same steps.

Studies of clinicians' information needs help us to understand the variability in diagnostic problem-solving among clinicians. Osheroff, Forsythe, and colleagues[4,5] used participant observation, a standard anthropological technique, to identify and classify information needs during the practice of medicine in an academic health center. They identified three components of "comprehensive information needs": (1) currently satisfied information needs (information recognized as relevant to a question and already known to the clinician); (2) consciously recognized information needs (information recognized by the clinician as important to know to solve the problem, but which is not known by the clinician); and (3) unrecognized information needs (information that is important for the clinician to know to solve a problem at hand, but is not recognized as being important by the clinician). Failure to detect a diagnostic problem at all would fall into the latter category. Different clinicians will experience different diagnostic problems within the same patient case, based on each clinician's varying knowledge of the patient and unique personal store of general medical knowledge. Osheroff and Forsythe noted the difficulty people and machines have in tailoring general medical knowledge to specific clinical cases. There may be a wealth of information in a patient's inpatient and outpatient records, and also a large medical literature describing causes of the patient's problems. The challenge is to quickly and efficiently reconcile one body of information with the other.[1,4] Clinical diagnostic decision support systems (CDDSS) can potentially facilitate that reconciliation. A CDDSS can be defined as:

> a computer-based algorithm that assists a clinician with one
> or more component steps of the diagnostic process [Definition 4].

While clinicians may have differing conceptions of what they mean by diagnosis, the definitions embodied in CDDSS are even more varied. CDDSS users are often slow to recognize that each system functionally defines diagnosis as the set of tasks that it can perform. Experienced users often become familiar with using CDDSS as tools to supplement, rather than replace their own diagnostic capabilities. Untrained CDDSS users have preconceived unrealistic expectations that engender subsequent frustration. Naïve users view diagnosis on their own terms, based on their own experiences, and expect diagnostic decision support systems to behave in a familiar manner. For example, it is unreasonable to expect that a CDDSS can solve a vague problem with minimal input, or that CDDSS can assist clinicians in understanding how an illness has affected the patient's lifestyle. Conversely, system developers sometimes create useful diagnostic tools that provide capabilities outside the experience of human diagnosticians. For example, the Relationships function of R-QMR* (a CDDSS), takes as input up to ten findings that the clinician-user would like to

---

* In this chapter, R-QMR refers to the research version of QMR, the CDDSS developed by Miller, Masarie and Myers.[6] The commercial version of QMR, marketed by First DataBank, while initially identical to R-QMR in 1990, has developed independently of R-QMR since that time.

explain as the key or "pivotal" findings from a diagnostically challenging case, and produces as output a rank-ordered list of "disease complexes" that each explain all of the input findings.[7] Each disease complex is made up of from 1 to 4 interrelated disorders (e.g., disease A predisposing to disease B and causing disease C). Because busy clinicians can spare little free time for extraneous activities, user training for CDDSS is extremely critical, and must address the potential cognitive mismatch between user expectations and system capabilities.

An important concept related to the use of CDDSS is understanding that the problem to be solved originates in the mind of the clinician-user. The diagnostic problem cannot be defined in an absolute sense, for example, by an arbitrary set of input findings selected from a case. The CDDSS analog of the metaphysical question, "if a tree falls in a forest in the absence of people, will there be a sound?" is "if clinical findings are extracted from a patient case in the absence of a query from a clinician caring for the patient (or someone asked to function with that mindset), is there a diagnostic problem to be solved, or can there be a 'correct' answer?" There is only one way that the findings of a case, in isolation, can define a diagnostic problem; that is when the diagnostic problem is the global one, i.e., the CDDSS, through its own initiative, is expected to take all the steps in the diagnostic process required to explain all patient findings through establishing new diagnoses (or unresolved differential diagnoses if there is not a solution). It is rare in clinical practice to encounter the "global" diagnostic problem. Clinicians usually complete a portion of the evaluation process before they encounter difficulty, and correspondingly, once they overcome the difficulty, they are usually capable of completing the evaluation without further assistance. While early CDDSS developers often assumed the only problem worth solving was the global diagnostic problem, emphasis over the last decade has shifted to helping clinicians with problems they encounter during individual steps in the diagnostic process. This has led to the demise of the "Greek Oracle" model where the CDDSS was expected to take all of the patient's findings and come up with "the answer." Current CDDSS models assume that the user will interact with the CDDSS in an iterative fashion, selectively entering patient information and using the CDDSS output to assist with the problems encountered in the diagnostic process.[8]

In order to interact optimally with the CDDSS, the users need to understand the assumptions built into the system. As noted previously, each CDDSS functionally defines diagnosis as the tasks it can perform (or assist users in performing). The subtle nature of underlying assumptions that system developers incorporate into CDDSS can be deceptive to users. For example, one of the most well-known diagnostic systems is the Bayesian program for diagnosis of acute abdominal pain developed by de Dombal and colleagues.[9,10] As it was originally developed, the system's goal, not stated explicitly, was to discriminate between surgical and nonsurgical causes of acute abdominal pain, in order to help triage patients in an emergency room (or similar) setting. A limited number of explicit diagnoses are supported by the system, all of which except "nonspecific abdominal pain" were surgical disorders or potentially surgically treated disorders (such as acute appendicitis, acute pancreatitis, and acute diverticulitis). The performance of the system was evaluated in multi-center studies[10] and shown to be exemplary with respect to the circumstances for which it was designed. However, naïve users generically relying on de Dombal's system to help with the diagnosis of all patients presenting with acute abdominal pain would be disappointed. There is a high potential for errors in caring for such patients if the clinician-users do not supplement system output with their own knowledge. The system could not properly diagnose patients presenting acute intermittent porphyria, lead poisoning, early T10 dermatome herpes zoster, or familial Mediterranean fever. Even when the system performs optimally, all these conditions would be labeled as "nonspecific abdominal pain."

The utility of making specific diagnoses lies in the selection of effective therapies, making accurate prognoses, and providing detailed explanations.[1] In some situations, it is not necessary to arrive at an exact diagnosis in order to fulfill one or more of these objectives. Treatment is often initiated before an exact diagnosis is made. Furthermore, the utility of making certain diagnoses is debatable, especially if there is a small probability of effective treatment. For instance, labeling a patient as having "obesity" does not flatter the patient, and even worse, may cause the clinician to do more harm than good. Good documentation exists in the medical literature that once a patient reaches approximately twice their ideal body weight, the patient's metabolism and psychology related to eating changes[11] so that the prognosis of dieting down to the ideal body weight and staying there is approximately equal to the survival rate for gastric carcinoma at five years. Resorting to "off-the-shelf", nonprescription, potentially harmful therapies such as liquid protein diets, unsupervised prolonged fasting, or prescribed amphetamines carries more harm than benefit, yet desperate patients and physicians sometimes resort to such approaches.

The cost of eliciting all possible patient data is potentially staggering—temporally, economically and ethically, since there are real risks of morbidity and/or mortality associated with many diagnostic procedures such as liver biopsy or cardiac catheterization. Given the impossibility and impracticality of gathering every conceivable piece of diagnostic information with respect to each patient, the "art" of diagnosis lies in the ability of the diagnostician to carefully evoke enough relevant information to justify all important and ultimately correct diagnoses in each case, and to initiate therapies at appropriate points during the evaluation.[2] The knowledge of how to "work up" the patient depends critically on the ability to evoke history, symptoms, and physical examination findings, concurrently with the ability to generate diagnostic hypotheses that suggest how to further refine or pursue the findings already elicited, or to pursue completely different additional findings. In addition, this must be done in a compassionate and cost-effective manner.[2]

HUMAN DIAGNOSTIC REASONING

Diagnostic reasoning involves diverse cognitive activities including: information gathering, pattern recognition, problem solving, decision making, judgment under uncertainty, and empathy. Large amounts of highly organized knowledge are necessary to function in this relatively unstructured cognitive domain. Our knowledge of human diagnostic reasoning is based on generic psychological experiments about reasoning, and on direct studies of the diagnostic process itself. Relevant principles of human problem-solving behavior have been unveiled through focused studies examining constrained problem spaces such as chess-playing and cryptoarithmetic.[12] Such studies have documented that experts recognize patterns of activity within a domain at an integrated, higher level ("chunking") than novices. Additional psychological experiments about judgments made under uncertainty[13] have provided insights into individuals' imperfect semiquantitative reasoning skills.

To investigate the complex intellectual task of clinical diagnosis, many researchers[14,15] have used behavioral methods that combine protocol analysis with introspection. Researchers record clinicians as they think aloud while performing specified cognitive tasks related to diagnosis (including normal clinical activities). Post facto, the clinicians themselves, or others, are asked to interpret the motives, knowledge, diagnostic hypotheses and strategies involved in the recorded sessions. However, there is no proof that the stories constructed by experts to explain their diagnostic reasoning correspond to the actual reasoning methods they use subconsciously.

Most models of diagnostic reasoning include the following elements: the activation of working hypotheses, the testing of these hypotheses, the acquisition and interpretation of additional information, and confirming, rejecting, or adding of new hypotheses as information is gathered over time. Working hypotheses are generated early in the process of information gathering, at a time when only few facts are known about the patient.[14,15] Only a limited number of these hypotheses, rarely more than five, are entertained simultaneously, probably because of the limited capacity of human short term memory.[16] Early hypothesis generation is probably accomplished through some form of pattern recognition, with experts more capable of applying compiled knowledge and experiences than novices. Comparing clinical reasoning in novices and experts, Evans and Patel[17] showed that experts rarely rely directly on causal reasoning and knowledge of basic sciences, except when reasoning outside their domain of expertise.

As noted by Pople and others,[18] clinical diagnosis fits Simon's criteria for being an ill-structured problem.[19] Simon gave as an example of an ill-structured problem, the task an architect faces in creatively designing a new house "from scratch"—the realm of possible solutions encompasses a great variety of applicable methods and a broad set of alternative outcomes. As summarized by Pople, Simon observed that ill-structured problems can be solved by splitting the problem into smaller, well-defined subtasks that are each more easily accomplished.[18]

In clinical diagnosis, early hypothesis generation helps to constrain reasoning to "high yield" areas, and permits the use of heuristic methods to further elucidate a solution.[20] Studies have shown that most clinicians employ the hypothetico-deductive method after early hypothesis generation.[14,15] Data are collected with a view to their usefulness in refining, rejecting or substituting for the original set of hypotheses. In the setting of clinicopathological exercises, Eddy and Clanton[21] showed that identification of a pivotal finding is often used to simplify the diagnostic problem, and to narrow the focus to a limited set of hypotheses. Kassirer and Gorry[15] described the "process of case building", where hypotheses are evaluated against the model of a disease entity using techniques that can be emulated in computers using Bayes' rule, Boolean algebra or template matching (see chapter 2 for an explanation of these terms). They also recognized that heuristic methods are commonly used to confirm, eliminate, discriminate or explore hypotheses. Weed[22] and Hurst and Walker[23] suggested that clinical problem-solving can be approached by splitting complex, composite problems into relatively independent, discrete "problem areas". With respect to diagnosis, Pople observed that separating complex differential diagnoses into problem areas allows diagnosticians to apply additional powerful reasoning heuristics. They can assume that the differential diagnosis list within a problem area contains mutually exclusive hypotheses, and that the list can be made to be exhaustive (i.e., complete)—so that it is assured that the correct diagnosis is on the list for the problem area, and that only one diagnosis on the list is the correct one.[18]

Kassirer has identified three abstract categories of human diagnostic reasoning strategies: probabilistic, causal and deterministic.[24] Formal models for each type of reasoning have been developed, most often separately from observational studies on how actual reasoning occurs. Probabilistic models such as Brunswik's lens model[25] and Bayesian[26,27] approaches, as well as decision analysis[28,29] define statistical associations between clinical variables and use mathematical models to compute optimal decisions. While it is clear that diagnosticians consider prevalence and other probabilistic concepts during their reasoning,[14,15] observational and experimental studies show that humans are not intuitively good statisticians.[13,30] Human problem-solvers tend to rely on judgmental heuristics. Experiments document that humans improperly evaluate subjective probabilities, misuse prior probabilities, and fail to recognize important phenomena, such as the regression towards the mean. While there has been some evidence that humans have more difficulty reasoning with probabilities than they do understanding the concepts which underlie them,[31] they also demonstrate other reasoning errors such as reluctance to revise opinions when presented with data that do not fit with working hypotheses when the data's diagnostic significance is properly understood.[13,30]

Models of causal (pathophysiological) reasoning, such as those developed by Feinstein[32,33] in the 1970s, establish cause-and-effect relations between clinical variables within anatomic, physiologic and biochemical representations of the reality. Although causal inferences (reasoning from causes to consequences) can be viewed as the inverse of diagnostic inferences (reasoning from consequences to causes), studies have shown that when making judgments under uncertainty, humans assign greater impact to causal rather than diagnostic data of equal informative weight, and commonly make over-confident predictions when dealing with highly uncertain models.[13] Causal, pathophysiological reasoning uses shared, global, patient-independent knowledge,[33] and provides an efficient means of verifying and explaining diagnostic hypotheses. However, it is not clear how much causal reasoning is actually used in early hypothesis generation and other stages of nonverbalized diagnostic reasoning. As noted earlier, observational studies indicate that experts tend to employ causal, pathophysiological reasoning only when faced with problems outside the realm of their expertise, or highly atypical problems, or when they are asked to explain their reasoning to others.[5]

In deterministic models, production rules, i.e., specifying appropriate actions in response to certain conditions, are used to represent the basic building blocks of human problem-solving. Such if-then rules representing compiled knowledge can be expressed in the form of branching-logic flow-charts and clinical algorithms for nonexperts to follow. However, production rules do not deal effectively with uncertainty,[34] which is a disadvantage in clinical practice, where uncertainty is a common feature.

The late M. Scott Blois, a great philosopher-informatician-clinician, used a funnel to illustrate the spectrum of clinical judgment.[35] Consideration of patients' ill-structured problems, including undifferentiated concerns and vague complaints, occurs at the wide end of the funnel. Focused decisions in response to specific clinical questions (e.g., choosing an antibiotic to treat the bacteria isolated as the cause of a pneumonia) were represented at the narrow end. This model is consistent with Simon's view of how humans solve ill-structured problems.[18] Blois noted that decision support systems were best applied toward the narrow end of the funnel, since circumscribed, well-structured problems are encountered there. Those problems are more amenable to solution through application of computational models of cognitive skills, requiring only focused and specific knowledge. On the other hand, at the open end of the funnel, one has to deal with common-sense knowledge and the general scope of ordinary human judgment in order to make meaningful progress, and few computer-based systems (other than those for record-keeping) are applicable.

HISTORICAL SURVEY OF CDDSS

The majority of important concepts related to current CDDSS were developed and presented in the literature prior to 1976. In a comprehensive 1979 review of reasoning strategies employed by early CDDSS, Shortliffe, Buchanan and Feigenbaum identified the following classes of CDDSS: clinical algorithms, clinical databanks that include analytical functions, mathematical pathophysiological models, pattern recognition systems, Bayesian statistical systems, decision-analytical systems, and symbolic reasoning (sometimes called "expert" systems).[36] This section, without being comprehensive, will describe how some of the early pioneering efforts led to many classes of systems present today.

The many types of CDDSS correspond to the large number of clinical domains to which diagnostic reasoning can be applied, to the multiple steps of diagnostic reasoning described above and to the variety of difficulties that diagnosticians may encounter at each step. When health care informatics researchers come upon the term "clinical diagnostic decision-support systems", many think primarily of general-purpose, broad-spectrum consultation systems.[1] However, definitions 1 to 3 in the section on definitions of diagnosis form the basis for the broad spectrum of diagnostic systems actually encountered. In a sense, definition 1, diagnosis as interpretation of raw observations, is potentially recursive as it defines successively more complex classes of diagnostic tools. Low-level diagnostic labels placed on "raw" observations can be used as input into second-level diagnostic systems that produce higher-level labels that are then used at progressively higher levels.

There are systems for general diagnosis (no matter how broad or narrow their application domains), and systems for diagnosis in specialized domains such as interpretation of ECG tracings.[37] The general notion of CDDSS conveyed in the biomedical literature some-times overlooks specialized, focused, yet highly successful medical device-associated diagnostic systems. Some simple CDDSS help to interpret blood gas results, assist in categorizing diagnostic possibili-ties based on the output of serum protein electrophoresis devices, or aid in the interpretation of standardized pulmonary function tests. CDDSS for cytological recognition and classification have found suc-cessful application in devices such as automated differential blood count analyzers and systems to analyze Papanicolaou smears.[1] Small, focused CDDSS are the most widely used form of diagnostic decision support programs, and their use will grow as they are coupled with other automated medical devices.[1]

In their classical paper published in 1959, Ledley and Lusted[26] observed that physicians have an imperfect knowledge of how they solve diagnostic problems. Ledley and Lusted detailed the principles underlying work on Bayesian and decision-analytic diagnostic sys-tems that has been carried out over subsequent decades. They stated that both logic (as embodied in set theory and Boolean algebra) and probabilistic reasoning (as embodied in Bayes' rule) were essential components of medical reasoning. Ledley and Lusted mentioned the importance of protocol analysis in understanding human diagnostic reasoning. They stated that they had reviewed how physicians solve *New England Journal of Medicine* CPC (clinicopathological confer-ence) cases as the foundation for their work on diagnostic computer systems. Both for practical reasons and for philosophical reasons, much work on CDDSS has focused on the differences between logical de-ductive systems and probabilistic systems. Chapter 2 describes these approaches in more detail. What follows is a description of how CDDSS have embodied these reasoning principles.

Logical systems, based on "discriminating questions" to distin-guish among mutually exclusive alternatives, have played an impor-tant role since the pioneering work by Bleich and his colleagues[38] on acid-base and electrolytes. To this day, such systems are applicable to narrow domains, especially those where it is fairly certain that only one disorder is present. When users of a branching logic system in-correctly answer one of the questions posed by the system, they may find themselves "out on a limb" with no way to recover except by start-ing over from the beginning; the likelihood of such problems increases when multiple independent disease processes interact in the patient.

Thus, ideal application areas are those where detailed knowledge of pathophysiology or extensive epidemiological data make it possible to identify parameters useful for dividing diagnostic sets into nonintersecting subsets based on specific characteristics.

Bayes' rule is applicable to larger domains. Warner and colleagues in 1960-61 developed one of the first medical application systems based on Bayes' rule. In their original contribution,[27] they discussed the independence assumption required among diagnoses and among findings by the most commonly employed Bayesian applications, and proposed a method for eliminating the influence of redundant findings. They obtained the probabilities used in the diagnosis of congenital heart diseases from literature review, from their own series of over 1000 cases, and from experts' estimates based on knowledge of pathophysiology. Warner et al. observed how diagnostic systems can be very sensitive to false positive findings, and to errors in the system's database. The importance of obtaining accurate data from the user was emphasized. In their evaluation of their system's performance, it was pointed out the need for an independent "gold standard" against which the performance of the system could be judged. In the evaluation of their system, they used cardiac catheterization data and/or anatomical (postmortem) data to confirm the actual patient diagnoses. Warner et al. have continued to develop and refine models for Bayesian diagnosis over the years.[1]

In 1968, Gorry and Barnett developed a model for sequential Bayesian diagnosis.[39] The first practical Bayesian system, and one of the first CDDSS to be utilized at widespread clinical sites, was the system for diagnosis of acute abdominal pain developed by de Dombal and colleagues.[1,9] A large number of groups have subsequently developed, implemented, and refined Bayesian methods for diagnostic decision-making, and a wave of enthusiasm surrounds current work on Bayesian belief networks for clinical diagnosis.[1] Probabilistic systems have played and will continue to play an important role in CDDSS development.

An additional alternative exists to categorical (predicate calculus)[40] and probabilistic reasoning, combining features of both, but retaining a fundamental difference. That alternative is heuristic reasoning, reasoning based on empirical rules-of-thumb. The HEME program for diagnosis of hematological disorders was one of the earliest systems to employ heuristics and also one of the first systems to use, in effect, criteria tables for diagnosis of disease states. It was developed initially by Lipkin, Hardy, Engle and their colleagues in the late 1950s.[1,41-43] Programs which heuristically match terminology from stored descriptions of disease states to lexical descriptions of patient cases are similar conceptually to HEME. The CONSIDER program developed by Lindberg et al.[44] and the RECONSIDER program developed by Blois and his colleagues[45] used heuristic lexical matching techniques to identify diseases in CMIT, a manual of diseases compiled and previously maintained by the American Medical Association. More recently, the EXPERT system shell developed by Weiss and Kulikowski[46] has been used extensively in developing systems that utilize criteria tables, including AI/Rheum[47-48] for diagnosis of rheumatological disorders, as well as others.

G. Anthony Gorry was an enlightened pioneer in the development of heuristic diagnostic systems that employ symbolic reasoning. In a classical paper in 1968, Gorry[49] outlined the general principles underlying expert system approaches to medical diagnosis that were subsequently developed in the 1970s and 1980s. Gorry proposed a formal definition of the diagnostic problem. In a visionary manner, he analyzed the relationships among a generic inference function (used to generate diagnoses from observed findings), a generic test-selection function that dynamically selects the best test to order (in terms of cost and information content), and a pattern-sorting function that is capable of determining if competing diagnoses are members of the same "problem area" (i.e., whether diagnostic hypotheses should be considered together because they are related to pathology in the same organ system). He pointed out the difference between the information value, the economic cost, and the morbidity or mortality risk of performing tests; discussed the cost of misdiagnosis of serious, life-threatening or disabling disorders; noted the potential influence of "red herring" findings on diagnostic systems; described the "multiple diagnosis" problem faced by systems when patients have more than one disease; and suggested that the knowledge bases underlying diagnostic systems could be used to generate simulated cases to test the diagnostic systems.

Gorry's schemata represent the intellectual ancestors of a diverse group of medical diagnostic systems, including, among others, PIP (the Present Illness Program) developed by Pauker et al., MEDITEL for adult illnesses which was developed by Waxman and Worley from an earlier pediatric version, Internist-I developed by Pople, Myers and Miller, QMR, developed by Miller, Masarie and Myers, DXplain, developed by Barnett and colleagues, Iliad, developed by Warner and colleagues, and a large number of other systems.[1,50-56]

Shortliffe introduced the clinical application of rule-based expert systems for diagnosis and therapy through his development of MYCIN[1,57] in 1973-1976. MYCIN used backward chaining through its rule base to collect information to identify the organism(s) causing bacteremia or meningitis in patients (see discussion of backward and forward chaining in chapter 2). A large number of rule-based CDDSS have been developed over the years, but most rule-based CDDSS have been devoted to narrow application areas due to the extreme complexity of maintaining rule-based systems with more than a few thousand rules.[1]

With the advent of the microcomputer came a change in philosophy in regard to the development of CDDSS. For example, the style of diagnostic consultation in the original 1974 Internist-I program treated the physician as unable to solve a diagnostic problem. The model assumed that the physician would transfer all historical information, physical examination findings, and laboratory data to the Internist-I expert diagnostic consultant program. The physician's subsequent role was that of a passive observer, answering yes or no to questions generated by Internist-I. Ultimately, the omniscient Greek Oracle (consultant program) was supposed to provide the correct diagnoses and explain its reasoning. By the late 1980s and early 1990s, developers abandoned the "Greek Oracle" model[8] of diagnostic decision support. Encouraged by the critiquing model developed by Perry Miller[1,58] and his colleagues, recent CDDSS developers have as an objective to create a mutually beneficial system that takes advantage of the strengths of both the user's knowledge and the system's abilities. The goal is to improve performance of both the user and the machine over their native (unassisted) states.

Several innovative techniques have been added in the 1980s and 1990s to previous models for computer-assisted medical diagnosis. The trend has been to develop more formal models that add mathematical rigor to the successful but more arbitrary heuristic explorations of the 1970s and early 1980s. However, there are tradeoffs involved in formal mathematical models, often related to available data quality, which in many ways make them heuristic as well.[59]

Systems based on fuzzy set theory and Bayesian belief networks were developed to overcome limitations of heuristic and simple Bayesian models.[1] Reggia, Nau and Wang[1,60] developed set covering models as a formalization of ad hoc problem-area formation (partitioning) schemes, such as that developed by Pople for Internist-I.[61]

Neural networks represent an entirely new approach to medical diagnosis, although the weights learned by simple one-layer networks may be analogous or identical to Bayesian probabilities.[1] Problems with neural networks include selecting the best topology, preventing overtraining and undertraining, and determining what cases to use for training. The more complex a neural network is (number of input and output nodes, number of hidden layers), the greater the need for a large number of appropriate training cases. Often large epidemiologically controlled patient data sets are not available. There is a tendency among some developers to resort to simulation techniques to generate training cases. Use of "artificial" cases to train neural networks may lead to sub-optimal performance on real cases. Chapters 2 and 7 describe the models mentioned above in more detail.

DEVELOPING, IMPLEMENTING, EVALUATING AND MAINTAINING CDDSS

For any CDDSS to achieve success, it must complete a number of stages of development.[2,62] To begin with, a CDDSS should be developed to meet documented information needs.[4,5,63] Developers must perform a clinical needs assessment to determine the utility of the proposed system, and the frequency with which it might be used in various real-world settings. Clinical systems should not be developed simply because someone wants to test an exciting new computational algorithm. The rule, "if it's not broke, don't fix it", applies to the development of CDDSS as well as other aspects of technology. Developers must carefully define the scope and nature of the process to be automated. They must also understand the process to be automated well enough to reduce the process to an algorithm. All systems, especially CDDSS, have boundaries (both in domain coverage and algorithm robustness) beyond which the systems often fail. Developers must understand these limits and make users aware of them. Each algorithm must be studied to determine the ways in which it might fail, both due to inherent limitations and due to flaws that might occur during the process of implementation.[2]

Developers and interested third parties must evaluate any automated system carefully, initially "in vitro" (outside of the patient care arena, with no risks to patients), and once warranted, in vivo (prospectively, on the front lines of actual patient care delivery) in order to determine if the automated system improves or promotes important outcomes that are not possible with the pre-existing manual system.[64] Finally, developers and users must demonstrate the practical utility of the system by showing that clinicians can adopt it for productive daily use.[2] A potentially great system that is not used cannot have a beneficial impact on clinical outcomes. Unfortunately, few, if any, of the existing clinical decision support systems have yet fulfilled these criteria.

There are a number of problems that have limited the ultimate success of CDDSS to date. These include: difficulties with domain selection and knowledge base construction and maintenance; problems with the diagnostic algorithms and user interfaces; the problem of system evolution, including evaluation, testing and quality control; issues related to machine interfaces, and clinical vocabularies; and legal and ethical issues. These issues are discussed below and are also addressed in more detail in later chapters.

CLINICAL DOMAIN SELECTION

CDDSS domain selection is often problematic. Substantial clinical domains must be chosen in order to avoid creating "toy" systems. However, construction of knowledge bases to support substantial CDDSS can require dozens of person-years of effort in broad domains such as general internal medicine. To date, although most large medical knowledge bases have at least initially been created in the academic environment, many projects do not have adequate funding to sustain such activity over time.[65] Availability of adequate domain expertise is also a problem. Clinical collaborators generally earn their wages through patient care or research, and sustaining high-level input from individuals with adequate clinical expertise can be difficult in the face of real-world demands. Commercial vendors must hire an adequate and well-qualified staff of physicians in order to maintain medical knowledge bases. However, the income generated through the sale of CDDSS programs is limited by the number of users who purchase a program or its updates, so that scaling up a CDDSS maintenance department can be difficult.

Different problems affect CDDSS with narrow domains. One problem is garnering an adequate audience. The CASNET system was an exemplary prototypic system for reasoning pathophysiologically about the diagnosis and therapy of glaucoma.[66] It typifies a problem that can occur with successful experimental expert systems—the persons most likely to require a specialized system's use in clinical medicine are the domain experts whose knowledge was used to develop the system. The persons who routinely diagnose and treat glaucoma are ophthalmologists, who are by definition Board-certified specialists in the domain of ophthalmology. The program, in effect, preaches to the choir. It is more difficult for an automated system to provide marginal benefit to experts in that speciality than to primary care providers, but generalists are unlikely to use a system with very narrow functioning. A program like the CASNET system must be extremely robust, and provide more than one kind of service (e.g., it should have integrated record-management and other functions) in order for it to find use in clinical practice.

KNOWLEDGE BASE CONSTRUCTION AND MAINTENANCE

Knowledge base maintenance is critical to the clinical validity of a CDDSS.[1] Yet, it is hard to judge when new clinical knowledge becomes an established "fact". The first reports of new clinical discoveries in highly regarded medical journals must await confirmation by other groups over time before their content can be added to a medical knowledge base. The nosological labels used in diagnosis reflect the current level of scientific understanding of pathophysiology and disease, and may change over time without the patient or the patient's illness per se changing.[1] For example, changes occur in how a label is applied when the "gold standard" for making a diagnosis shifts from a pathological biopsy result to an abnormal serological test—patients with earlier, previously unrecognized forms of the illness may be labeled as having the disease. Corresponding changes must be made to keep a CDDSS knowledge base up-to-date.

Knowledge base construction must be a scientifically reproducible process that can be accomplished by qualified individuals at any site.[67] Knowledge base construction should be clinically grounded, based on "absolute" clinical knowledge whenever possible. Attempts to "tune" the CDDSS knowledge base to improve performance on a given case or group of cases should be strongly discouraged, unless such tuning has an objective basis, such as information culled from the medical literature. If the process of knowledge base construction is highly dependent on a single individual, or can only be carried out at a single institution, then the survival of that system over time is in jeopardy. While much of the glamour of computer-based diagnostic systems lies in the computer algorithms and interfaces, the long-term value and viability of a system depends on the quality, accuracy and timeliness of its knowledge base.[1]

Even initially successful CDDSS cannot survive unless the medical knowledge bases supporting them are kept current. This can require Herculean efforts. Shortliffe's MYCIN program[57] was developed as a research project to demonstrate the applicability of rule-based expert systems to clinical medicine. MYCIN was a brilliant, pioneering effort in this regard. The evaluation of MYCIN in the late 1970s by Yu and colleagues demonstrated that the program could perform at the expert level on challenging cases.[68] But MYCIN was never placed into routine clinical use, nor was an effort made to update its knowledge base over time. After 1979, lack of maintenance caused its antibiotic therapy knowledge base to become out of date.

CDDSS DIAGNOSTIC ALGORITHMS AND USER INTERFACES

Just as computer-based implementation of many complex algorithms involves making tradeoffs between space (memory) and time (CPU cycles), development of real-world diagnostic systems involves a constant balancing of theory (model complexity) and practicality (ability to construct and maintain adequate medical databases or knowledge bases, and ability to create systems which respond to users' needs in an acceptably short time interval).[59] We may understand, in theory, how to develop systems that take into account gradations of symptoms, the degree of uncertainty in the patient and/or physician-user regarding a finding, the severity of each illness under consideration, the pathophysiological mechanisms of disease, and/or the time course of illnesses. Such complexities may ultimately be required to make actual systems work reliably. However, it is not yet practical to build such complex, broad-based systems for patient care. The effort required to build and maintain superficial knowledge bases is measured in dozens of person-years of effort, and more complex knowledge bases are likely to require an order of magnitude greater effort.[1]

Although some people believe that the computer will eventually replace the physician,[69] that position is not very tenable. A clinician cannot convey his or her complete understanding of an involved patient case to a computer program. One can never assume that a computer program "knows" all that needs to be known about the patient case, no matter how much time and effort is spent on data input into the computer system. As a result, the clinician-user who directly evaluated the patient must be considered to be the definitive source of information about the patient during the entire course of any computer-based consultation.[2] In addition, the highly skilled health care practitioner, who understands the patient as a person, possesses the most important intellect to be employed during a consultation. That user should intellectually control the process of computer-based consultation. CDDSS must be designed to permit users to apply individual tools to assist with the sequence of steps in the diagnostic process in the sequence that the user prefers at the time, not in an arbitrary sequence selected by the CDDSS algorithm.

All CDDSS, and especially narrowly focused ones, face the "critical mass" problem. Few clinicians are likely to purchase and install office computer systems solely to run one application. The number of narrow CDDSS that could be useful in the setting of a primary care practitioner's office is potentially measured in tens or hundreds. Yet few computer-literate individuals learn how to successfully operate more than a dozen applications. Until there is a standard, integrated environment and user interface that allows smooth transition among dedicated applications, CDDSS are not likely to be used heavily. It is possible that the Internet, with a common user interface across multiple hardware platforms, will evolve to be the integrated environment required. However, current limitations of such interfaces leave this an open question. Systems must provide flexible environments that adapt to the user's needs and problems, rather than providing an interface that is inflexible and which penalizes the user for deviating from the normal order of system operation. It must be easy to move from one program function to another if it is common for the health care user to do so on their own mentally. Transitions must be facilitated when frequent patterns of usage emerge.

CDDSS Testing, Evaluation and Quality Control

System evaluation in biomedical informatics should take place as an ongoing, strategically planned process, not as a single event or small number of episodes.[61,64] Complex software systems and accepted medical practices both evolve rapidly, so evaluators and readers of evaluations face moving targets. As previously noted, systems are of value only when they help users to solve users' problems. Users, not systems, characterize and solve clinical diagnostic problems. The ultimate unit of evaluation should be whether the user plus the system is better than the unaided user with respect to a specified task or problem (usually one generated by the user).

It is extremely important during system development to conduct informal "formative" type evaluations. As a part of this process, new cases must be analyzed with the CDDSS on a regular (e.g., weekly) basis. After each failure of the CDDSS to make a "correct" diagnosis, careful analysis of both the system's knowledge base and diagnostic algorithms must be carried out. Both the information in the knowledge base on the "correct" diagnosis, and the information on any diagnoses offered in error, must be reviewed and potentially updated. In addition, periodic re-running of previous series of test cases should be done on an annual (or similar basis), to verify that there has not been significant "drift" in either the knowledge base or the diagnostic program that would influence the system's abilities.

Formal evaluations of CDDSS should take into account the following four perspectives: (1) appropriate evaluation design; (2) specification of criteria for determining CDDSS efficacy in the evaluation; (3) evaluation of the boundaries or limitations of the CDDSS; and (4) identification of potential reasons for "lack of system effect."[64] Each of these issues is discussed below.

Appropriate Evaluation Design

Evaluation plans should be appropriate for the information needs being addressed, the level of system maturity, and users' intended form of CDDSS usage (or specific system function evaluated).[62,64] The same CDDSS may serve as an electronic textbook for one user, a diagnostic checklist generator for another user, a consultant to determine the next useful step in a specific patient's evaluation for a third user, and a tool to critique/reinforce the users' own pre-existing hypotheses for a fourth user. Each system function would require a different form of evaluation whenever anticipated user benefits depend on which system function is used. Evaluations should clearly state which user objective is being studied, and which of the available system functions are relevant to that objective.

In 1994, Berner[70] and colleagues evaluated the ability of several systems to generate first-pass differential diagnoses from a fixed set of input findings. These findings were not generated by everyday clinical users, but came from written case summaries of real patient data. That approach was dictated by the desire to standardize system inputs and outputs for purposes of multi-system use. The primary goal of Berner et al. was to develop methods and metrics that would characterize aspects of system performance in a manner useful for rationally comparing different systems and their functions. All of the systems in that study were capable of generating questions to further refine the initial differential diagnoses, which is the intended mode of clinical use for such systems. Because that study was not intended to produce a definitive rating or comparison of the systems themselves, the involved systems were not placed in the hands of end-users, nor were the systems used in a manner to address common end-user needs. Even though the evaluation did not examine this capability, the methods used by Berner were sound. Generating a first-pass differential diagnosis is a good initial step, but subsequent evidence-gathering, reflection, and refinement are required.

There are important questions that must be answered in the evaluation. Are the problems ones that clinical users generate during clinical practice, or artificial problems generated by the study design team? Is the case material accurately based on actual patient cases? Note that there can be no truly verifiable diagnosis when artificial, manually-constructed or computer-generated cases are used. Are the evaluation subjects clinical users whose participation occurs in the clinical context of caring for the patients used as "test cases?" Are clinical users evaluating abstracts of cases they have never seen or are nonclinical personnel evaluating abstracted clinical cases using computer systems? Are users free to use all system components in whatever manner they choose, or is it likely that the study design will constrain users to exercise only limited components of the system? The answers to these questions will determine the generalizability of the results of the evaluation.

Specification of Criteria for Determining CDDSS Efficacy in the Evaluation

Evaluations must determine if the criteria for "successful" system performance are similar to what clinical practitioners would require during actual practice. Diagnosis itself, or more properly, "diagnostic benefit", must be defined in such contexts. Similarly, what it means to establish a diagnosis must be carefully defined. For example, it is not adequate to accept hospital discharge diagnoses at face value as a "gold standard", since discharge diagnoses are not of uniform quality—they have been documented to be influenced by physician competency, coding errors, and economic pressures. Furthermore, some discharge diagnoses may be "active" (undiagnosed at admission and related to the patient's reason for hospitalization), while others may be relevant but inactive. Criteria for the establishment of a "gold standard" diagnosis should be stated prospectively, before beginning data collection.

Evaluation of the Boundaries or Limitations of the CDDSS

A system may fail when presented with cases outside its knowledge base domain, but if an evaluation only uses cases from within that domain, this failure may never be identified. The limits of a system's knowledge base are a concern because patients do not accurately triage themselves to present to the most appropriate specialists. For instance, as discussed earlier, de Dombal's abdominal pain system performed very well when used by surgeons to determine if patients presenting with abdominal pain required surgery. However, a patient with atypical appendicitis may present to an internist, and a patient with abdominal pain due to lead poisoning may first see a surgeon.

Identification of Potential Reasons for "Lack of System Effect"

CDDSS operate within a system that not only includes the CDDSS itself, but also the user and the health care environment in which the user practices. A model of all of the possible influences on the evaluation outcomes would include CDDSS-related factors (knowledge base inadequacies, inadequate synonyms within vocabularies, faulty algorithms, etc.), user-related factors (lack of training or experience with the system, failure to use or understand certain system functions, lack of medical knowledge or clinical expertise, etc.)

and external variables (lack of available gold standards, failure of patients or clinicians to follow-up during study period). It is important to recognize that studies that focus on one aspect of system function may have to make compromises with respect to other system or user-related factors in order to have an interpretable result. Additionally, in any CDDSS evaluation, the user's ability to generate meaningful input into the system, and the system's ability to respond to variable quality of input from different users, is an important concern.

Evaluations of CDDSS must each take a standard objective (which may be only one component of system function) and measure how effectively the system enhances users' performances—using a study design that incorporates the most appropriate and rigorous methodology relative to the stage of system development. The ultimate clinical end-user of a given CDDSS must determine if published evaluation studies examine the system's function in the manner that the user intends to use it. This is analogous to a practitioner determining if a given clinical trial (of an intervention) is relevant to a specific patient by matching the given patient's characteristics to the study's inclusion and exclusion criteria, population demographics, and the patient's tolerance for the proposed forms of therapy as compared to alternatives. The reporting of an individual "negative study" of system performance should not, as it often does now, carry the implication that the system is globally suboptimal. A negative result for one system function does not mean that for the same system, some users cannot derive significant benefits for other system functions. Similarly, complete evaluation of a system over time should examine basic components—e.g., the knowledge base, ability to generate reasonable differential diagnoses, ability to critique diagnoses, etc.—as well as clinical functionality—e.g., can novice users after standard training successfully employ the system to solve problems that they might not otherwise solve as efficiently or completely. The field of CDDSS evaluation will become mature only when clinical system users regularly derive the same benefit from published CDDSS evaluations as they do from evaluations of more standard clinical interventions.

CDDSS INTERFACE AND VOCABULARY ISSUES

A critical issue for the success of large-scale, generic CDDSS is their environment. Paradoxically, small, limited, "niche" systems will be adopted and used by the focused community for which they are intended, while physicians in general medical practice, for whom the large-scale systems are intended, may not have need for diagnostic assistance on a frequent enough basis to justify purchase of one or more such systems. Therefore, it is common wisdom that CDDSS are most likely to succeed if they can be integrated into a clinical environment so that patient data capture is already performed by automated laboratory and/or hospital information systems. In such an environment, the physician will not have to manually enter all of a patient's data in order to obtain a diagnostic consultation. However, it is not straightforward to transfer the information on a patient from a hospital information system to a diagnostic consultation system. If 100 hematocrits were measured during a patient's admission, which one(s) should be transferred to the consultation system—the mean, the extremes, or the value typical for a given time in a patient's illness? Should all findings be transferred to the consultation system, or only those findings relevant to the patient's current illness? These questions must be resolved by careful study before one can expect to obtain patient consultations routinely and automatically within the context of a hospital information system. Another reason for providing an integrated environment is that users will not use a system unless it is sufficiently convenient to do so. By integrating CDDSS into health care provider results reporting and order entry systems, the usual computer-free workflow processes of the clinician can be replaced with an environment conducive to accomplishing a number of computer-assisted clinical tasks, making it more likely that a CDDSS will be used.

Interfaces between automated systems are at times as important as the man-machine interface. Fundamental questions, such as the definition of diseases and of findings, limit our ability to combine data from the literature, from clinical databanks, from hospital information systems, and from individual experts' experiences in order to create CDDSS. Similar problems exist when trying to match the records from a given case (collected manually or taken from an electronic medical record) with a computer-based diagnostic system. A diagnostic system may embody different definitions for patient descriptors than those of the physician who evaluated the patient, even though the words used by each may be identical.

In order to facilitate data exchange among local and remote programs, it is mandatory to have a lexicon or interlingua which facilitates accurate and reliable transfer of information among systems which have different internal vocabularies (data dictionaries). The United States National Library of Medicine Unified Medical Language System (UMLS) project, which started in 1987 and continues through the present time, represents one such effort.[71]

LEGAL AND ETHICAL ISSUES

Proposals have been made for governmental agencies, such as the United States Food and Drug Administration (FDA), which oversees medical devices, to regulate use of clinical software programs such as CDDSS. These proposals include a variety of recommendations that manufacturers of such systems would be required to perform to guarantee that the systems would function per specifications.

There is debate about whether these consultation systems are actually devices in the same sense as other regulatable devices. In the past, governmental regulation has not been considered necessary when a licensed practitioner is the user of a CDDSS.[72] It would be both costly and difficult for the government to regulate CDDSS more directly, even if a decision were made to do so. For general CDDSS programs like Iliad, QMR, Meditel and DXplain, with hundreds to thousands of possible diagnoses represented in their knowledge bases,[70] conducting prospective clinical trials to demonstrate that the system worked for all ranges of diagnostic difficulty for a variety of patients with each diagnosis would require enrollment of huge numbers of patients and would cost millions of dollars.

Other approaches, such as a "software quality audit" to determine, prospectively, if a given software product has flaws, also would be clinically impractical. The clinician seeking help may have any of several dozen kinds of diagnostic problems in any given case. Unless it is known, for a given case, which kind of problem the practitioner will have, performing a software quality audit could not predict if the system would be useful.

Consider the dilemma the FDA or other responsible regulatory agency would face if it agreed to review situations when a user files a complaint. First, one must note that few patients undergo definitive enough diagnostic evaluations to make it possible to have a "gold standard" (certain) diagnosis. So if the doctor claims the program was wrong, a major question would be how governmental auditors would know what the actual "right" diagnosis was. Second, the reviewers would need to know all of the information that was knowable about the patient at the time the disputed diagnosis was offered. This could potentially violate patient confidentiality if the records were sent to outsiders for review. All sources of information about the patient would have to be audited, and this could become as difficult as evidence gathering in a malpractice trial. To complete the sort of audit described, the governmental agency would have to determine if the user had been appropriately trained and if the user used the program correctly. Unless the program had an internally stored complete audit trail of each session (down to the level of saving each keystroke the user typed), the auditors might never be able to re-create the session in question. Also, the auditors would have to study whether the program's knowledge base was appropriate. Initial development of the R-QMR knowledge base at the University of Pittsburgh required an average of three person-weeks of a clinician's time which went into literature review of 50-150 primary articles about each disease, with additional time for synthesis and testing against cases of real patients with the disease. For an auditor to hire the required expertise to review this process for hundreds to thousands of diseases for each of the programs that it would have to review and subsequently monitor would be costly and cumbersome. The ultimate question, very difficult to answer, would be whether the original user in the case in question used the system in the best way possible for the given case. Making such a determination would require the governmental agency to become expert in the use of each CDDSS program. This could take up to several months of training and practice for a single auditor to become facile in the use of a single system. It would be difficult for a governmental agency to muster the necessary resources for even a small number of such complaints, let alone nationwide for multiple products with thousands of users. The complexity of these issues make it very difficult to formulate appropriate regulatory policy. In addition to legal issues concerning regulation, there are other legal and ethical issues relating to use of CDDSS that are discussed in chapter 9.

THE FUTURE OF CDDSS

It is relatively safe to predict that specialized, focused CDDSS will proliferate, and a sizable number of them will find widespread application.[1] As new medical devices are developed and older devices automated, CDDSS software which enhances the performance of the device, or helps users to interpret the output of the device, will become essential. Computerized ECG analysis, automated arterial blood gas interpretation, automated protein electrophoresis reports, and automated differential blood cell counters are but a few examples of such success at the present time.

The future of large-scale, "generic" diagnostic systems is hopeful, although less certain. As discussed in this and other chapters, a number of major challenges remain to be solved before CDDSS that address large medical problem domains can succeed over time. No matter what the level of use of large-scale, generic CDDSS in clinical practice, it is well established that such systems can play a valuable role in medical education.[1] The process of knowledge base construction, utilization of such knowledge bases for medical education in the form of patient case simulations, and the use of CDDSS have all been shown to be of educational value in a variety of institutional settings (see chapter 5).

In summary, the future of CDDSS appears to be bright. The number of researchers in the field is growing. The diversity of CDDSS is increasing. The number of commercial enterprises interested in CDDSS is expanding. Rapid improvements in computer technology continue to be made. A growing demand for cost-effective clinical information management, and the desire for better health care is sweeping the United States. All these factors will insure that new and productive CDDSS applications will be developed, evaluated and used.

REFERENCES

1. Miller RA. Medical diagnostic decision support systems—past, present, and future: a threaded bibliography and commentary. JAMIA 1994; 1:8-27.
2. Miller RA. Why the standard view is standard: people, not machines, understand patients' problems. J Med Philos 1990; 15:581-591.
3. Flexner SB, Stein J, eds. The Random House College Dictionary, Revised Edition. New York: Random House, Inc.,1988,366.
4. Osheroff JA, Forsythe DE, Buchanan BG et al. Physicians' information needs: an analysis of questions posed during clinical teaching in internal medicine. Ann Intern Med 1991; 114:576-581.

5. Forsythe DE, Buchanan BG, Osheroff JA et al. Expanding the concept of medical information: an observational study of physicians' information needs. Comput Biomed Res 1992; 25:181-200.
6. Miller R, Masarie FE, Myers J. Quick Medical Reference (QMR) for diagnostic assistance. MD Comput 1986; 3:34-48.
7. Miller RA, Masarie FE Jr. The quick medical reference (QMR) relationships function: description and evaluation of a simple, efficient "multiple diagnoses" algorithm. Medinfo 1992:512-518.
8. Miller RA, Masarie FE Jr. The demise of the "Greek Oracle" model for medical diagnosis systems. Methods Inf Med 1990; 29:1-2.
9. de Dombal FT, Leaper DJ, Horrocks JC et al. Human and computer-aided diagnosis of abdominal pain: further report with emphasis on performance of clinicians. Br Med J 1974; 1:376-380.
10. Adams ID, Chan M, Clifford PC et al. Computer aided diagnosis of acute abdominal pain: a multicentre study. Br Med J (Clin Res Ed) 1986; 293:800-804.
11. Rosenbaum M, Leibel RL, Hirsch J. Obesity. N Engl J Med 1997; 337:396-407.
12. Newell A, Simon HA. Human Problem Solving. Englewood Cliffs, NJ: Prentice Hall, 1972.
13. Kahneman D, Slovic P, Tversky A, eds. Judgment Under Uncertainty: Heuristics and Biases. Cambridge, UK: Cambridge University Press, 1982.
14. Elstein AS, Shulman LS, Sprafka SA. Medical problem solving: an analysis of clinical reasoning. Cambridge, MA: Harvard University Press, 1978.
15. Kassirer JP, Gorry GA. Clinical problem-solving—a behavioral analysis. Ann Intern Med 1978; 89:245-255.
16. Miller GA. The magical number seven, plus or minus two: some limits on our capacity for processing information. Psychol Rev 1956; 63:81-97.
17. Evans DA, Patel VL, eds. Cognitive Science in Medicine. Cambridge, MA: MIT Press, 1989.
18. Pople HE Jr. Heuristic methods for imposing structure on ill-structured problems: the structuring of medical diagnostics. In Szolovits P, ed. Artificial Intelligence in Medicine. AAAS Symposium Series. Boulder, CO: Westview Press. 1982, 119-190.
19. Simon HA. The structure of ill-structured problems. Artif Intell 1973; 4:181-201.
20. Miller RA, Pople HE Jr, Myers J. Internist-I, an experimental computer-based diagnostic consultant for general internal medicine. N Engl J Med 1982; 307:468-476.
21. Eddy DM, Clanton CH. The art of diagnosis: solving the clinicopathological conference. N Engl J Med 1982; 306:1263-1269.
22. Weed LL. Medical records that guide and teach. N Engl J Med 1968; 278:593-600 and 652-657.

23. Hurst JW, Walker HK, eds. The Problem-Oriented System. New York, NY: Medcom Learning Systems, 1972.
24. Kassirer JP. Diagnostic reasoning. Ann Intern Med 1989; 110:893-900.
25. Brunswik E. Representative design and probabilistic theory in a functional psychology. Psychol Rev 1955; 62:193-217.
26. Ledley RS, Lusted LB. Reasoning foundations of medical diagnosis. Science 1959; 130:9-21.
27. Warner HR, Toronto AF, Veasey LG et al. Mathematical approach to medical diagnosis. JAMA 1961; 177:75-81.
28. Raiffa H. Decision analysis. Reading, MA: Addison-Wesley Inc. 1970.
29. Pauker SG, Kassirer JP. Decision analysis. N Engl J Med 1987; 316:250-258.
30. Dawes RM, Faust D, Meehl PE. Clinical versus actuarial judgment. Science 1989; 243:1668-1674.
31. Gigerenzer G, Hoffrage U. How to improve Bayesian reasoning without instruction: frequency formats. Psychol Rev 1995; 102:684-704.
32. Feinstein AR. An analysis of diagnostic reasoning. I. The domains and disorders of clinical macrobiology. Yale J Biol Med 1973; 46:212-232.
33. Feinstein AR. An analysis of diagnostic reasoning. II. The strategy of intermediate decisions. Yale J Biol Med 1973; 46:264-283.
34. Horvitz EJ, Heckerman DE. The inconsistent use of measures of certainty in artificial intelligence research. In: Uncertainty in Artificial Intelligence, Vol 1. Amsterdam; New York: Elsevier Science, 1986, 137-151.
35. Blois MS. Clinical judgment and computers. N Engl J Med 1980; 303:192-197.
36. Shortliffe EH, Buchanan BG, Feigenbaum EA. Knowledge engineering for medical decision-making: a review of computer-based clinical decision aids. Proc IEEE 1979; 67:1207-1224.
37. Willems JL, Abreu-Lima C, Arnaud P et al. The diagnostic performance of computer programs for the interpretation of electrocardiograms. N Engl J Med 1991; 325:1767-1773.
38. Bleich HL. Computer evaluation of acid-base disorders. J Clin Invest 1969; 48:1689-1696.
39. Gorry GA, Barnett GO. Experience with a model of sequential diagnosis. Comput Biomed Res 1968; 1:490-507.
40. Szolovits P, Pauker SG. Categorical and probabilistic reasoning in medical diagnosis. Artif Intell 1978; 11:114-144.
41. Lipkin M, Hardy JD. Differential diagnosis of hematological diseases aided by mechanical correlation of data. Science 1957; 125:551-552.
42. Lipkin M, Hardy JD. Mechanical correlation of data in differential diagnosis of hematological diseases. JAMA 1958; 166:113-123.
43. Lipkin M, Engle Jr RL, Davis BJ et al. Digital computer as an aid to differential diagnosis. Arch Intern Med 1961; 108:124-140.

44. Lindberg DAB, Rowland LR, Buch CR Jr et al. CONSIDER: A computer program for medical instruction. Proc Ninth IBM Medical Symposium, 1968.
45. Nelson SJ, Blois MS, Tuttle MS et al. Evaluating RECONSIDER: a computer program for diagnostic prompting. J Med Sys 1985; 9:379-388.
46. Weiss S, Kulikowski CA. EXPERT: a system for developing consultation models. Proc Sixth Int Joint Conf Artif Intell 1979.
47. Lindberg DAB, Sharp GC, Kingsland LC et al. Computer based Rheumatology consultant. Medinfo 1980:1311-1315.
48. Moens HJ, van der Korst JK. Development and validation of a computer program using Bayes's theorem to support diagnosis of rheumatic disorders. Ann Rheum Dis 1992; 51:266-271.
49. Gorry A. Strategies for computer aided diagnosis. Math Biosci 1968; 2:293-318.
50. Pauker SG, Gorry GA, Kassirer JP et al. Towards the simulation of clinical cognition. Taking a present illness by computer. Am J Med 1976; 60:981-996.
51. Waxman HS, Worley WF. Computer-assisted adult medical diagnosis: subject review and evaluation of a new microcomputer-based system. Medicine 1990; 69:125-136.
52. Pople HE, Myers JD, Miller RA. DIALOG: A model of diagnostic logic for internal medicine. Proc Fourth Int Joint Conf Artif Intell 1975:848-855
53. First MB, Soffer LJ, Miller RA. QUICK (Quick Index to Caduceus Knowledge): Using the Internist-I/Caduceus knowledge base as an electronic textbook of medicine. Comput Biomed Res 1985; 18: 137-165.
54. Miller RA, McNeil MA, Challinor S et al. Status Report: The Internist-1 / Quick Medical Reference project. West J Med 1986; 145:816-822.
55. Hupp JA, Cimino JJ, Hoffer EF et al. DXplain—A computer-based diagnostic knowledge base. Medinfo 1986; 5:117-121.
56. Warner HR, Haug P, Bouhaddou O et al. ILIAD as an expert consultant to teach differential diagnosis. Proc Annu Symp Comput Appl Med Care 1987:371-376.
57. Shortliffe EH. Computer-Based Medical Consultations: MYCIN. New York, NY: Elsevier Computer Science Library, Artificial Intelligence Series, 1976.
58. Miller PL. A Critiquing Approach to Expert Computer Advice: ATTENDING. Boston: Pittman, 1984.
59. Aliferis CF, Miller RA. On the heuristic nature of medical decision-support systems. Methods Inf Med 1995; 34: 5-14.
60. Reggia JA, Nau DS, Wang PY. Diagnostic expert systems based on a set covering model. Internat J Man-Machine Stud 1983; 19:437-460.

61. Berman L, Miller RA. Problem area formation as an element of computer aided diagnosis: a comparison of two strategies within quick medical reference (QMR). Methods Inf Med 1991; 30:90-95.
62. Stead WW et al. Designing medical informatics research and library-resource projects to increase what is learned. JAMIA 1994; 1:28-34.
63. Covell DG, Uman GC, Manning PR. Information needs in office practice: are they being met? Ann Int Med 1985; 103:596-599.
64. Miller RA. Evaluating evaluations of medical diagnostic systems. JAMIA 1996; 3:429-431.
65. Yu VL. Conceptual obstacles in computerized medical diagnosis. J Med Phil 1983; 8:67-75.
66. Weiss S, Kulikowski CA, Safir A. Glaucoma consultation by computer. Comput Biol Med 1978; 8:24-40.
67. Giuse NB, Giuse DA, Miller RA et al. Evaluating consensus among physicians in medical knowledge base construction. Methods Inf Med 1993; 32:137-145.
68. Yu VL, Fagan LM, Wraith SM et al. Antimicrobial selection by computer: a blinded evaluation by infectious disease experts. JAMA 1979; 242:1279-1282.
69. Mazoue JG. Diagnosis without doctors. J Med Philos 1990; 15:559-579.
70. Berner ES, Webster GD, Shugerman AA et al. Performance of four computer-based diagnostic systems. N Engl J Med 1994; 330:1792-1796.
71. Lindberg DA, Humphreys BL, McCray AT. The Unified Medical Language System. Methods Inf Med 1993; 32:281-291.
72. Young FE. Validation of medical software: present policy of the Food and Drug Administration. Ann Intern Med 1987; 106:628-629.

CHAPTER 2

Mathematical Foundations of Decision Support Systems

S. Andrew Spooner

M any computer applications may be considered to be clinical decision support systems. Programs that perform MEDLINE searches or check drug interactions do support decisions, but they are not "clinical decision support systems" in the usual sense. What we usually mean by a clinical decision support system is a program that supports a reasoning task, carried out behind the scenes and based on clinical data. For example, a program that accepts thyroid panel results and generates a list of possible diagnoses is what we usually recognize as a clinical diagnostic decision support system (CDDSS). General purpose programs that accept clinical findings and generate diagnoses are the typical CDDSS. These programs employ numerical and logical techniques to convert clinical input into the kind of information that a physician might use in performing a diagnostic reasoning task. How these numerical techniques work is the subject of this chapter.

Essential to the understanding of CDDSS is familiarity with the basic principles of logic and probability. A brief review of these areas is offered first, followed by a description of a general model of CDDSS, which will help in understanding how some CDDSS perform reasoning tasks. Exceptions to the model will round out this discussion of the mathematical foundations of CDDSS.

REVIEW OF LOGIC AND PROBABILITY

Set Theory

A brief review of basic concepts in set theory is helpful in understanding logic, probability, and many other branches of mathematics. A *set* is a collection of unique objects. For example, the major Jones criteria[1] for rheumatic fever is a set:

Jones-Criteria-Major ={carditis, migratory polyarthritis, erythema marginatum, chorea, subcutaneous nodules}

Likewise, the minor criteria make a set:

Jones-Criteria-Minor = {fever, arthralgia, elevated acute phase reactants, prolonged P-R interval on electrocardiogram}

To complete our description of the Jones criteria, we need a third set:

Group-A-Strep-Evidence = {positive culture, positive rapid antigen, antibody rise or elevation}.

To apply the Jones criteria, one compares the patient's findings with the items in the various sets above. A patient is highly likely to have rheumatic fever if there is evidence of group A streptococcal infection and the patient has two major criteria or one major and two minor criteria.

Each *element* or *member* of the set is distinguishable from the others. A *subset* is any collection of elements of a known set. Using the first of the criteria above, a patient must have a subset of clinical findings containing at least two of the elements of Jones-Criteria-Major to meet the Jones criteria for rheumatic fever. If a patient has the clinical findings:

Findings ={migratory polyarthritis, chorea, subcutaneous nodules}

then we say that Findings is a subset of Jones-Criteria-Major, or, in set terminology:

Findings $\subseteq$ Jones-Criteria-Major

The *cardinality* or *size* of a set is simply the number of elements in the set. For our two examples, the cardinalities (written by placing a vertical bar before and after the symbol for the set) are:

|FINDINGS| = 3
|JONES-CRITERIA-MAJOR| = 5

The basic set operations are *intersection* and *union*. The intersection of two sets is the set of elements the two sets have in common. For example, if there is a patient with the following set of clinical findings:

CLINICAL-FINDINGS = {heart murmur, migratory polyarthritis, chorea, subcutaneous nodules, cough}

then the intersection of this set and JONES-CRITERIA-MAJOR is written:

CLINICAL-FINDINGS ∩ JONES-CRITERIA-MAJOR

It is easy to see that the intersection of these two sets is simply the set FINDINGS. The union of two sets is the set of all elements that belong to either set. Since, by definition, a set's elements must be distinguishable from one another, the set resulting from the union of our patient's findings and the Jones major criteria is written:

CLINICAL-FINDINGS ∪ JONES-CRITERIA-MAJOR = {heart murmur, migratory polyarthritis, chorea, subcutaneous nodules, cough, carditis, erythema marginatum, chorea}

Anyone who has done a MEDLINE search in which two sets of literature citations are combined has performed these set operations; the AND function in MEDLINE is like set intersection, and the OR function is like set union.

Diagnostic criteria like the Jones criteria are good examples of how sets can be used to represent diagnostic rules. The full Jones criteria, represented in set theoretical terminology, might read like this (assuming we have sets JONES-CRITERIA-MINOR and GROUP-A-STREP-EVIDENCE described at the beginning of this section):

If CLINICAL-FINDINGS is the set of a given patient's symptoms, signs, and laboratory test results, then the patient is highly likely to have rheumatic fever if either of two conditions are met:
1. |CLINICAL-FINDINGS ∩ JONES-CRITERIA-MAJOR| ≥ 2
and
|CLINICAL-FINDINGS ∩ GROUP-A-STREP-EVIDENCE| ≥1

2. |CLINICAL-FINDINGS ∩ JONES-CRITERIA-MAJOR| = 1
and
|CLINICAL-FINDINGS ∩ JONES-CRITERIA-MINOR| ≥ 2
and
|CLINICAL-FINDINGS ∩ GROUP-A-STREP-EVIDENCE| ≥1

There are other set operations besides union and intersection. For example, the phenomenon of *set covering* has application in decision making. A cover of a set is a set of subsets in which each element of the covered set appears at least once as a member of one of the sets in the cover set. An example makes this definition clearer. Suppose you were asked to recommend a list of antibiotics for your hospital's emergency department. Your objective is to stock the minimum number of antibiotics that will be effective for 95% of the pathogenic organisms you've found in cultures at your hospital. For the sake of simplicity, suppose that there are six pathogens, each designated by a letter, which account for 95% of the infections seen in your hospital. You might represent this set of pathogens as:

PATHOGENS = {A, B, C, D, E, F}

You have the following set of antibiotics from which to choose:

ANTIBIOTICS = {A-Cillin, B-Cillin, C-Cillin, D-Cillin, E-Cillin, F-Cillin}

Each antibiotic is described by the set of pathogens for which that antibiotic is effective.
Here is a list of your antibiotics, with their covered pathogen sets (each of which is a subset of PATHOGENS):

- A-Cillin = {A, C}
- B-Cillin = {A, B, E}
- C-Cillin = {C, D, E}
- D-Cillin = {F}
- E-Cillin = {B, D, F}
- F-Cillin = {E}

What you seek is a set cover of the set PATHOGENS; in other words, you want to pick a set of antibiotics which contains at least one antibiotic that is effective for each pathogen. It's clear that all six antibiotics taken together make a set cover, but your job is to find the minimum number of antibiotics that will get the job done. Casual inspection shows that the set {A-Cillin, E-Cillin, F-Cillin} does the job as a set cover, in that at least one antibiotic in that set is effective for each one of the pathogens in PATHOGENS.

There are many other set operations which can be applied to real-world decision problems, but the brief introduction presented here should suffice to illuminate the concepts presented in this book. Generally speaking, sets are used to formalize logical operations in a way that a machine—usually a computer—can understand.

Before we leave the topic of sets, fuzzy sets are worth a brief mention. Under conventional principles of set theory, an element is either a member of a set or it isn't. Heart murmur, for example, is definitely not a member of the set JONES-CRITERIA-MAJOR. Under *fuzzy set theory*, membership in a set is not an all-or-none phenomenon. In a fuzzy set, an element is a member of the set with a certain probability; e.g., cough is a member of the set COLD-SYMPTOMS with a probability of 80% (a 4 out of 5 chance). Fuzzy set theory has created new ways of looking at sets and new methods for applying set theory to solve decision-making problems: fuzzy logic.[2-3] Fuzzy logic has been used to tackle decision-making problems in which uncertainty plays a role.

BOOLEAN LOGIC

Anyone who has performed a search of the medical literature using the MEDLINE system has used logic. When referring to common logical operations like combining two sets of literature citations using AND or OR, we often refer to these operations as "Boolean" logic, in honor of George Boole (1815-1864), a British mathematics professor who published seminal works on formal logic. Indeed, MEDLINE is not a bad way to learn about Boolean algebra, since its connection to set theory is made so clear by the sets of literature citations that we manipulate in that system.

Suppose we have performed two literature searches. The result of one search, set A, represents all the literature citations in the MEDLINE database that relate to rheumatoid arthritis. Set B consists of all the literature citations on immune globulin. By asking the MEDLINE program to give us a new set that is the result of combining A and B using the AND operator, we have a new set, C, that contains literature citations on the use of immune globulin in rheumatoid arthritis. When we combine two sets of citations using the AND function of our MEDLINE program, we are asking the computer to give us all citations that appear in both sets. This corresponds roughly to the English use of the word *and*.

The word *or* in Boolean logic has a slightly different meaning than in English. In everyday usage, *or* usually has an exclusive meaning; the statement "You may opt for chemotherapy or radiation therapy" usually means that one may have one or the other therapy, but not both. The Boolean OR is different. If one were to perform another pair of MEDLINE searches, this time for all articles that have asthma as a keyword (set A) and those that mention "reactive airway disease" in the text of the abstract (set B), one could combine sets A and B with the OR function to get a comprehensive set of citations on asthma. Because the OR function takes all citations that appear in one or both of sets A and B, the OR function is said to be *inclusive*.

There are other Boolean operators, like XOR (exclusive OR: "either A or B but not both") and NAND ("A and not B"), but AND and OR are the basic operators with which we are familiar.

How is Boolean logic used in CDDSS? The mathematical subjects of statement logic and predicate logic give us formal definitions of how statements can be combined to produce new conclusions. For example, consider the following statements:

1. Urine cultures with colony counts of 10,000 or more are considered positive, if they are obtained by bladder catheterization.
2. This patient's urine culture shows more than 10,000 colonies of *E. coli*.
3. All patients with positive urine cultures should be treated for urinary tract infections.

The statements can be combined intuitively, without the use of formal mathematics, into the conclusion:

This patient needs to be treated for a UTI.

The logic that gave us the conclusion so easily comes from our medical intuition, but computers have no intuition. They must be programmed to generate even the most obvious conclusions. To understand logic as it is implemented on a computer, one must understand the basics of predicate logic and deductive reasoning.

The above example about UTIs is a sloppy instance of a syllogism. A syllogism is a form of deductive reasoning consisting of a major premise, a minor premise, and a conclusion. The premises are combined, using rules of predicate logic, into a conclusion. For example, a syllogism in a ventilator management decision support system might be:

Major Premise: All blood gas determinations that show carbon dioxide to be abnormally low indicate an over-ventilated patient.

Minor Premise: The current patient's carbon dioxide is abnormally low.

Conclusion: Therefore, the current patient is overventilated.

Again, this conclusion is obvious, but by representing the above syllogism by symbols, where the symbol Low-CO_2 represents the state of abnormally low carbon dioxide and the symbol OVERVENTILATED represents the state of an overventilated patient, the syllogism looks more computer-friendly:

Major Premise: Low-CO_2 $\Rightarrow$ OVERVENTILATED
Minor Premise: Low-CO_2
Conclusion: OVERVENTILATED

Extending this example, suppose we have another statement in our CDDSS that overventilation should cause a high rate alarm to sound (we can represent this by the symbol HIGH-RATE-ALARM, then we can construct the syllogism:

Major Premise: Low-CO_2 $\Rightarrow$ Overventilated
Minor Premise: Overventilated $\Rightarrow$ High-Rate-Alarm
Conclusion: Low-CO_2 $\Rightarrow$ High-Rate-Alarm

Thus, we have generated a new rule for the system, where the intermediate state of overventilation is bypassed. This simplification of two rules into a new one may or may not help our understanding of the system, but the results the system gives are the same: A low carbon dioxide value sets off the high rate alarm. One can imagine how large sets of rules can be combined with each other to reduce complex reasoning tasks to simple ones.

The syllogism above is an example of rule chaining, where two rules are chained together to form a new conclusion. Specifically, the simple system outlined above is a *forward-chaining deduction system*, because the system starts with *if* statements and moves to a *then* statement. In real life, though, we often start with the "then" portion of a logical rule. For instance, consider the clinical rule:

> If your patient has asthma, then give an influenza immunization each fall.

There are many other rules in real clinical practice with the same "then" portion ("give a flu vaccine"). The question a clinician might ask is not "Does this patient have asthma? If so, I should give a flu shot" but more likely the question would be simply "Does this patient need a flu shot?" We start with the "then" portion of this set of flu shot rules. A *backward-chaining deduction system* does this–it starts with the "then" end of a set of rules and works backwards to answer questions based on its rule set. In the flu shot example, a backward-chaining system would start with the "Does this patient need a flu shot" question and immediately learn that the diagnosis of asthma would cause this rule to be satisfied. The system might then ask the user or query a clinical database about the presence of this diagnosis.

An example of a backward-chaining deduction system in medicine is the MYCIN system developed at Stanford.[4] MYCIN's domain was the selection of antibiotics for the treatment of bacterial infections based on clinical and microbiological information. An example of a forward-chaining system in medicine is Germwatcher developed at Barnes Hospital in St. Louis.[5] Germwatcher uses as its rules the Centers for Disease Control and Prevention's National Nosocomial Infections Surveillance System.[6] Using a computer program which helps implement a forward-chaining reasoning system called CLIPS (C Language Integrated Production System, Software Technology Branch, National Aeronautics and Space Administration, Johnson Space Center, Houston, TX) expert system shell Germwatcher works in a large hospital microbiology laboratory to identify nosocomial infections early from culture data.

CDDSS that use logic like the simple ventilator-management system above have limited application, since the range of truth encompassed by this logical system includes only true (e.g., the High Rate alarm needs to be sounded) or false (e.g., the High Rate alarm does not need to be sounded). Not many applications in medicine can be reduced to such simple truths. There may be situations where the High Rate might not always have to be sounded for a low carbon dioxide (e.g., for a head injury patient who needs a low carbon dioxide to preserve cerebral blood flow). To accommodate these situations it would be helpful if the response from the system were something like "the high rate alarm should probably be sounded." Such a system would then need to be able to handle probabilities as well as certainties, which most CDDSS do. MYCIN, for example, reports its conclusions in terms of their likelihood. The next section covers basic concepts of probability.

PROBABILITY

Everyday medical practice contains many examples of probability. We often use words such as probably, unlikely, certainly, or almost certainly in all conversations with patients. We only rarely attach numbers to these terms, but computerized systems must use some numerical representation of likelihood in order to combine statements into conclusions.

Probability is represented numerically by a number between 0 and 1. Statements with a probability of 0 are false. Statements with a probability of 1 are true. Most statements from real life fall somewhere in the middle. A probability of 0.5 or 50% are just as likely to be true as false. A round, opacified area seen in the lungs on a chest radiograph is probably pneumonia; one might assign a probability of 0.8 or 80% (a 4 in 5 chance) to this statement. Based on the high probability of pneumonia, one might elect to treat this condition without performing further testing—a lung biopsy, perhaps—that would increase the probability of pneumonia to greater than 80%. We are accustomed to accepting the fact that our diagnoses have a certain probability of being wrong, so we counsel patients about what to do in the event (we might use the term "unlikely event") that things don't work out in the expected way.

Probabilities can be combined to yield new probabilities.
For example, the two statements:

Pr(diabetes) = 0.6
Pr(hypertension) = 0.3

means that the probability of diabetes is 0.6 or 60% (3 in 5 chance), and the probability of hypertension is 0.3 or 30% (3 in 10 chance). We have not specified the clinical context of these statements, but suppose these probabilities applied to a particular population. Suppose further that the two conditions are independent; that is, the likelihood of patients having one disease is unaffected by whether they have the other (not always a safe assumption!). If we then want to know what the probability of finding a patient in our specified population with both diseases, we simply multiply the two probabilities (0.6 and 0.3) to get 0.18 or 18%. If the two clinical conditions are not independent, e.g., pulmonary emphysema and lung cancer–then we cannot combine the probabilities in such a simple, multiplicative manner. This is much like the AND function in MEDLINE or the intersection function as applied to sets.

The familiar "OR" function from our MEDLINE program also has a mathematical meaning in combining probabilities. If we wanted to know how many patients in the above example had diabetes *or* hypertension (remember: this would also include those with both diseases in the usual mathematical sense of *or*), we would compute:

Pr(diabetes OR hypertension) = Pr(diabetes) +
Pr(hypertension) − Pr(diabetes AND hypertension)

The last term in the above equation we already know to be $0.6 \times 0.3 = 0.18$, so:

Pr(diabetes OR hypertension) = 0.6 + 0.3 − 0.18 = 0.72.

Conditional probability is another type of probability often used in medicine. A conditional probability is the probability of an event (or the probability of the truth of a statement) *given the occurrence of another event* (or the truth of another statement). The most familiar case of conditional probability in medicine arises in the interpretation of diagnostic tests. For example, the probability of pneumonia given a round density on chest radiograph is what we need to know in interpreting that diagnostic test if it is positive. In mathematical notation, this conditional probability is written this way:

Pr(Pneumonia | Round Density on CXR)

One reads this notation, "The probability of pneumonia given a round density on chest radiograph." This notation is convenient in the explanation of Bayes' rule, which is the cornerstone of the logic in many decision support systems.

BAYES' RULE

If we have a patient with jaundice, how likely is it that he has hepatitis? Written another way, we seek to learn:

Pr(hepatitis | jaundice)

which is read as "the probability of hepatitis given the presence of jaundice." we may not have this probability at our fingertips, but we might be able to find a slightly different probability more easily:

Pr(jaundice | hepatitis)

which is, simply, the probability of jaundice given the presence of hepatitls. The latter probability could be found by studying a series of patients with proven hepatitis (it would be easy to get this data by looking up diagnosis codes in the medical records department) and computing the percentage of these patients who present with jaundice. However, this does not directly answer our original question. Bayes' rule allows us to compute the probability we *really* want— Pr(hepatitis | jaundice)—with the help of the more readily available number Pr(jaundice | hepatitis). Bayes' rule[7] is simply this:

$$Pr(\text{hepatitis} \mid \text{jaundice}) = \frac{Pr(\text{hepatitis}) \times Pr(\text{jaundice} \mid \text{hepatitis})}{Pr(\text{jaundice})}$$

Notice that to solve this equation, we need not only Pr(jaundice | hepatitis), but Pr(hepatitis)–the probability of hepatitis independent of any given symptom–and Pr(jaundice)–the probability of jaundice independent of any particular disease. These two independent probabilities are called *prior probabilities*, since they are the probabilities prior to the consideration of other factors.

The derivation of Bayes' rule is very simple. We already know that the probability of any two events occurring simultaneously is simply the product of their individual probabilities. For example, the joint probability we already computed of diabetes and hypertension in a hypothetical population was:

$$Pr(\text{diabetes AND hypertension}) = Pr(\text{diabetes}) \times Pr(\text{hypertension}) = 0.6 \times 0.3 = 0.18.$$

We were free to multiply these together, because in our hypothetical population, the likelihood of one disease occurring in an individual was independent of the other. In other words:

$$Pr(\text{hypertension}) = Pr(\text{hypertension} \mid \text{diabetes})$$

and

$$Pr(\text{diabetes}) = Pr(\text{diabetes} \mid \text{hypertension}).$$

In this population, one's chance of having one disease is unaffected by the presence of the other disease.

In medicine, we are often faced with the question of the likelihood of two interrelated events occurring simultaneously in a patient. The case of a diagnostic test and the disease it is supposed to test for is a good example: What is the probability of an abnormal chest radiograph and pneumonia occurring in the same patient simultaneously? This question asks for this probability:

$$Pr(\text{pneumonia AND abnormal CXR})$$

Can't we simply find out what the incidence of pneumonia in the population is, and multiply it by the incidence of abnormal chest radiographs in the population? A moment's reflection should show that this simple calculation is not sufficient. For example, if the incidence of pneumonia is 1 in 1000, and the incidence of abnormal chest radiograph is 1 in 100, then the erroneous probability would be computed:

WRONG: $Pr(\text{pneumonia AND abnormal CXR}) =$

$$\frac{1}{1000} \times \frac{1}{100} = 0.00001 = 0.001\%$$

This does not fit with our clinical intuition very well, since we know that people with pneumonia tend to have abnormal chest films. Our intuition says that the probability of the two events occurring together should be pretty close to the probability of having pneumonia alone, since a majority of those patients will have abnormal chest films. What we *really* need to compute is this:

$$Pr(\text{pneumonia AND abnormal CXR}) = Pr(\text{pneumonia}) \times Pr(\text{abnormal CXR} \mid \text{pneumonia})$$

This is the probability of pneumonia multiplied by the probability of an abnormal chest radiograph given that pneumonia exists. If we take $Pr(\text{abnormal CXR} \mid \text{pneumonia})$ to be 90%, then the computation matches our intuition much better.

In general, for any two events A and B:

$$Pr(A \text{ AND } B) = Pr(A) \times Pr(B \mid A)$$

and

$$Pr(B \text{ AND } A) = Pr(B) \times Pr(A \mid B)$$

But since $Pr(A \text{ AND } B)$ must surely equal $Pr(B \text{ AND } A)$, we can say that the right hand sides of the equations above are equal to each other:

$$Pr(A) \times Pr(B \mid A) = Pr(B) \times Pr(A \mid B)$$

Rearranging this equation, we have Bayes' Rule:

$$Pr(A \mid B) = \frac{Pr(A) \times Pr(B \mid A)}{Pr(B)}$$

At an intuitive level, we use Bayes' rule when making seat-of-the-pants estimates of disease probability in patients. For example, if we designate hepatitis by A, and jaundice by B and there were an ongoing epidemic of hepatitis (i.e., $Pr(A)$ was high) then our index of suspicion for hepatitis in a jaundiced person would be increased. Likewise, if the likelihood of jaundice due to other causes was high (i.e., $Pr(B)$ was high) then our estimation of the probability of hepatitis as a specific diagnosis would be lowered. Similarly, if jaundice were pathognomonic of hepatitis (i.e., $Pr(A|B)$ was 1 or near to it), then our hepatitis diagnosis would be greatly increased. By using numerical estimates of the probability of diseases, findings and conditional probabilities, Bayes' rule can help make medical decisions.

One might imagine a simple CDDSS in which one enters a single symptom and receives the probability of the presence of a disease given that symptom. A problem arises when one wishes to get disease probabilities given multiple symptoms. The number of data points needed to do Bayesian calculations on multiple simultaneous symptoms is huge. For example, in a system which handles only single symptoms, if one had a database of 1000 symptoms and 200 diseases, one would need to create $1000 \times 200 = 200,000$ conditional probabilities, 1000 symptom probabilities, and 200 disease probabilities, for a total of about 200,000 numbers. Since most of these numbers are zero (many symptoms are unrelated to many diseases) this may be a reasonable number of numbers to collect into a knowledge base. When one starts considering the probabilities needed to do computations on two simultaneous symptoms, this number climbs from 200,000 to about 200,000,000! If one wanted to design a system that could handle the very realistic situation of 5 or 6 simultaneous symptoms, estimating the number of numbers needed to support the calculation would be intractable. Modifying the system to handle multiple simultaneous "diseases" adds even more to the complexity. Only after making the simplifying assumption that most disease findings are independent of one another[8] do many CDDSS use Bayesian approaches. One such system, Iliad,[9] profitably employs this assumption.

INFORMAL LOGIC

Even if we create a reasoning system that follows all the rules of logic and probability, it would be difficult to come up with all the numbers that must be assigned to each event in even a small clinical database. Many successful CDDSS have circumvented this difficulty by employing informal rules of logic to accomplish the reasoning task without creating an intractable data-gathering task. In the early development of one of the most famous CDDSS, MYCIN,[4,10] the creators of the system developed their own logic system (heuristic) that made intuitive sense. This system employed "certainty factors" which ranged from –1 (false) to +1 (true). A certainty factor of zero indicated no belief in either direction in the statement's veracity. In combining several statements with the AND function into a single combined statement in MYCIN, one simply takes the minimum certainty factor of all the statements as the certainty factor of the combined statement. This makes a certain intuitive sense: we cannot be any more certain of an AND statement than we are of the least certain part. Later development of the MYCIN project showed a sound probabilistic basis for the certainty factor rules, but the point here is that sometimes cutting mathematical corners can still yield a useful system. In both the QMR[11] and DXplain[12] CDDSS, there is a database of diseases and findings (a finding is an item from the history, physical examination, laboratory data, or radiographic data). Each disease is defined by a particular set of findings. Each disease-finding relationship is assigned a frequency (of the finding among people with the disease) and an evoking strength (of how strongly a finding would evoke the possibility of a disease) on an ordinal scale (1-5 for frequency; 0-5 for evoking strength). These two factors make intuitive sense, and the system works, but the manipulation of these factors within these systems is very different from the formal algebra of logic and probability.

THE GENERAL MODEL OF DIAGNOSTIC DECISION SUPPORT SYSTEMS

There are similarities between physician and CDDSS reasoning, although a CDDSS might arrive at a similar conclusion to a physician without employing the same model of reasoning. Physicians do use some probabilistic information when they make decisions. For instance, a physician might make a diagnosis of influenza more often during the winter when influenza was more prevalent (probable) than in the summer. However, physicians use this information in informal ways; in other words, they do not actually use numbers in formulas to make diagnostic decisions.[13-15] Another feature of real-life clinical decision making is that physicians do not require complete information to make a decision. Most doctors are comfortable making decisions based on incomplete or contradictory information.[16] In contrast, CDDSS rely on well-defined numerical techniques to do their reasoning, and they do require sufficient information to complete their formulae. While physicians can fall back on their knowledge of pathophysiology, CDDSS are not well suited to situations in which hard data are unknown. To understand how these systems operate, and under what conditions they are best used, it is important to appreciate a general model of CDDSS.

Figure 2.1 shows a general model of CDDSS. There is input to the system and output from it. The CDDSS has a reasoning (inference) engine and a knowledge base. Understanding these basic

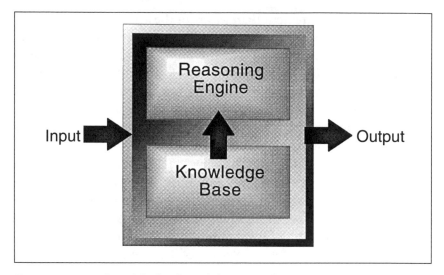

Fig. 2.1. A general model of a clinical diagnostic decision support system.

components provides a useful framework for understanding most CDDSS and their limitations. There are systems which do not follow this model which will be discussed later in this chapter.

The user supplies input appropriate to the system (i.e. terms from the system's controlled vocabulary to represent clinical data), and the system supplies output (e.g., a differential diagnosis). The reasoning engine applies formal or informal rules of logic to the input, and often relies on additional facts encoded in the system's knowledge base. The knowledge base is the compilation of the relationships between all of the diseases in the system and their associated manifestations (e.g., signs, symptoms, laboratory and radiographic tests). Maintaining the knowledge base in such systems is the most significant bottleneck in the maintenance of such systems, since the knowledge base needs to be expanded and updated as medical knowledge grows.

INPUT

The manner in which clinical information is entered into the CDDSS (user interface) varies from system to system, but most systems require the user to select terms from its specialized, controlled vocabulary. Comprehension of natural language has been an elusive goal in the development of CDDSS. While it would be highly desirable to be able to speak or type the query "What are the diagnostic possibilities for a four-year-old child with joint swelling and fever for a month," most who have used such systems are accustomed to the task of reformatting this question in terms the particular CDDSS can understand. We might, for example, break the above query into components:

- Age: 4 years
- Gender: unspecified
- Symptom: joint swelling
- Duration: one month
- Time course: unknown

This breakdown of the original query might work on one system, but another system might demand that we break it down another way:

- Age: less than 12 years
- Finding: arthritis

Notice that the second description describes the age in vague terms, and it forces us to eschew joint swelling for the more specific term arthritis (usually defined as joint pain, redness, warmth, and swelling). In the vocabulary of the program the age of four years (as opposed to 10 years) is unimportant, and joint swelling without other signs of inflammation is undefined.

Any physician who has assigned diagnostic and procedural codes in billing systems understands the limitations of controlled vocabularies. In a CDDSS, it is common for the user's input to be restricted to a finite set of terms and modifiers. How well the system works in a given clinical situation may depend on how well the system's vocabulary matches the terms the clinician uses. CDDSS take a variety of terms, called findings, which encompass items from the medical history, physical examination, laboratory results, and other pieces of clinical information. What constitutes a valid finding in a given program is entirely up to the program; there is no "standard" set of findings for all CDDSS. For general purpose CDDSS, items from the history and physical examination are going to be the findings. In specialized domains, e.g., an arterial-blood-gas expert system, the input vocabulary will be entirely different and much more restrictive.

Entering "chest pain" as a finding in a CDDSS may be insufficient to capture the essence of the symptom. "Chest pain radiating to the left arm" may be sufficient, but usually there are pertinent temporal factors related to symptoms that are difficult to express in a controlled vocabulary. For example, "sudden onset, 20 minutes ago, of chest pain radiating to the left arm" has a very different meaning from "five-year history of continuous chest pain radiating to the left arm." While CDDSS often include a vocabulary of severity and location modifiers, temporal modifiers are more difficult to build into a system, since minute changes in the timing of onset and duration can make a big difference in the conclusion the system reaches. Some CDDSS make simplifying assumptions about broad categories of timing (acute, sub-acute, chronic) to aid in the temporal description of findings. Although users may experience frustration in being unable to enter temporal information, the research is equivocal on its impact.

One solution to the problem of temporal modeling in CDDSS is to use an explicit model of time, in which the user is asked to specify intervals and points in time, along with temporal relationships between events (e.g., event A occurred before event B), in order to drive a temporal reasoning process within the CDDSS. Clearly, this complicates the matter of entering data (to say nothing of programming the system!). A simpler approach is to model time implicitly. In implicit time,[17] temporal information is built into the data input elements of the CDDSS; no special temporal reasoning procedures are required. For example, one input item could be "history of recent exposure to Strep." By joining the concept "history of" with the concept of a particular bacterial pathogen, one successfully abstracts the temporal nature of this finding, which would be pertinent in the diagnosis of rheumatic fever or post-streptococcal glomerulonephritis. Note that no explicit definition of "recent" is part of this representation; if for some reason one needed to distinguish infection 2 weeks ago from infection 3 months ago, this abstraction would not suffice. Thus, there is a disadvantage to this simplification. Nonetheless, CDDSS which use implicit temporal abstractions seem to perform well for time-sensitive clinical cases.

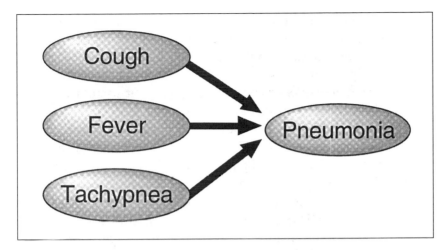

Fig. 2.2. A Bayesian network for the diagnosis of pneumonia.

INFERENCE ENGINE

There are many ways of programming an inference engine. The inference engine is the portion of the CDDSS that combines the input and other data according to some logical scheme for output. Users of the system do not usually know—or need to know—how the engine works to achieve the results.

One such scheme for an inference engine is the Bayesian network. Recall that Bayes' rule helps us express conditional probabilities—the likelihood of one event given that another has occurred. A Bayesian network is a way to put Bayes' rule to work by laying out graphically which events influence the likelihood of occurrence of other events. Figure 2.2 shows a Bayesian network for the diagnosis of pneumonia.

The arrows in the diagram indicate all of the conditional relationships between findings and diagnoses. Note that the symptoms listed are not necessarily independent; since febrile patients are often tachypneic, even in the absence of lung disease, one cannot say the two are as independent as Bayesian reasoning requires. Conceptually, this network simply states that the diagnosis of pneumonia is supported by the presence of three symptoms. The strength of association—that is, how strongly pneumonia is suggested by each of the three symptoms—varies with each symptom-disease pairing. By "activating" all three nodes (cough, fever, and tachypnea) the probability of pneumonia is maximized. Of course, each of these three nodes might be tied to other disease states in the database (like lung cancer or upper respiratory infection).

Bayesian networks can be complex, but their usefulness comes from their ability to represent knowledge in an intuitively appealing way. Inference engines that operate on the basis of a network simply adjust probabilities based on simple mathematical relationships between nodes in the network. Iliad,[9] a general CDDSS, is one such program which is built on Bayesian reasoning, and whose reasoning engine can be described as a Bayesian network. Mammonet[18] is a mammography CDDSS built on a Bayesian network whose nodes include quality of the breast mass, age at menarche, age of the patient, type of calcification of the mass, and other findings apt to be present in the evaluation of a mammogram.

Production rule systems are another method of programming an inference engine. The rules of predicate logic dictate the functioning of such an engine as it combines statements to form new conclusions. MYCIN, described earlier, uses a production rule system. Production rules are an intuitively attractive way to start thinking about CDDSS, since so much of the care physicians give in daily practice follows certain well known rules (e.g., giving patients with asthma an influenza vaccine each year). Other CDDSS using production rules include IMM/Serve,[19] a rule-based immunization decision-making program accessible via the Internet at http://ycmi.med.yale.edu/immserve/ and Hepaxpert (MED-EXPERT Data Systems Ltd., Vienna, Austria) a rule-based hepatitis serology expert system available via the Internet at http://www.med-expert.co.at/hepax/welcome.htm.

An appealing solution to the problem of constructing inference engines in a clinical setting is to develop a cognitive model of actual clinical reasoning. In other words, one could study the reasoning that a physician uses and attempt to create a computerized version of that cognitive task. Workers in the field of artificial intelligence, in modeling human cognition, have developed the notion of "frames" or schemes as a reasonable cognitive model. A frame consists of a set of "slots" into which is fit details of a particular kind of information. For example, a disease frame may have a slot for etiologic agent and time course. Frames can be used to construct a semantic network model of the world, which may then be searched for answers to questions based on a particular situation. One such application of frames in medicine is the criterion-table method of diagnosing diseases like rheumatoid arthritis or Kawasaki disease. By applying a list of criteria, physicians can classify patients by diagnosis. The AI/Rheum system[20] employs this familiar device in an inference engine that can be used outside its original domain of rheumatologic diseases.

One important aspect of inference engines is their independence from their knowledge base. Since CDDSS take a great deal of time to develop, re-usability has been a focus of research.[21] Theoretically, one should be able to take any inference engine and apply it in any domain. In reality, a given inference engine is developed with a particular domain in mind and its use does not move from that domain.

KNOWLEDGE BASE

For CDDSS to work, they must possess some form of medical knowledge. Obviously, the method of encoding of this knowledge must match the inference engine design. For example, a CDDSS based on a Bayesian network must contain probabilities–prior, conditional, and posterior–of diseases and findings. A big obstacle to building such a knowledge base is that many relevant probabilities are not known. While the medical literature can surely help with this task and CDDSS developers use the literature to varying degrees in building their knowledge bases, knowledge base developers must resort to estimates of probabilities based on the clinical judgment of experts to fill in the needed numbers. Unfortunately, physicians can exhibit markedly variable behavior in supplying such numbers,[22] and probabilities can vary from situation to situation even with the same disease entities (e.g., variations in disease prevalence with different populations).

Once one creates a knowledge base and populates it with some amount of data, the next task is to create a way to maintain it. Since many CDDSS begin as funded academic research projects, it is no wonder that development of their knowledge bases often halts after the grant funds cease. Since knowledge base maintenance takes a tremendous amount of time, and since the market for CDDSS is rather small, many CDDSS become too expensive to maintain. The knowledge-acquisition bottleneck[23] has been recognized as a problem in CDDSS research.

OUTPUT

The output of CDDSS is usually in the form of a list of possibilities, ranked in some order of probability. Sometimes probability is not the only criterion on which results are evaluated; for example, in the DXplain output, diseases which are not necessarily very likely, but whose misdiagnosis would be catastrophic, are flagged with a special disease-importance tag to call attention to the possibility.[12] Very often, physicians are not interested in the most likely diagnosis from a CDDSS; for experienced physicians, the most likely diagnosis is obvious. It is the less likely diagnosis that one might fail to consider that interests physicians in CDDSS, yet clearly it is difficult to draw the line between the rare and the ultra-rare.

NON-KNOWLEDGE-BASED SYSTEMS

The systems discussed so far have been knowledge based in the sense that an expert must expressly encode medical knowledge into numerical form for the systems to work. The knowledge-based systems cannot simply "learn" how to do the reasoning task from modeling human experts; the human expert must put the knowledge into the system explicitly and directly.

NEURAL NETWORKS

There are systems which can learn from examples. Neural networks are the most widely recognized of these types of systems, and there are regular reports in the medical literature on their use in diverse fields.[24-27]

Artificial neural networks are constructed in a fashion similar to biological neural networks. Neuron bodies ("nodes") are connected to one another by axons and dendrites ("links"). Nodes may be turned on or off, just as a biological neuron can be in an activated or inactivated state. Activation of a node causes activation of a signal on a link. The effect of that signal depends on the weight assigned to that link. In most learning neural networks, some nodes are input nodes and some are output nodes. In the CDDSS context, the input nodes would be findings and the output nodes would be possible diseases. To understand how a neural network might work, consider the problem of determining whether a person with a sore throat has streptococcal infection (as opposed to a harmless viral infection). There are many input nodes to this decision, and perhaps two output nodes:

Strep infection and viral infection. By presenting to a neural network many thousands of cases of sore throat (where the outcome is known), the neural network would "learn," for example, that the presence of cough decreases the likelihood of Strep, and the height of fever increases this likelihood.

The appealing feature of neural networks—and what separates this technique from other methods of discovering relationships among data, like logistic regression—is the ability of the system to learn over time. A neural network changes its behavior based on previous patterns. In a domain where the relationship between findings and diseases might change, like infectious disease surveillance, this changing behavior can be desirable. Another desirable feature of neural networks is the lack of necessity to understand complex relationships between input variables; the network learns these relationships as it changes the links between its nodes. This is the principal difference between neural networks and Bayesian networks; in the latter, one explicitly constructs the network based on one's knowledge of pathophysiology and known probabilities. With neural networks, the links are established as the network is developed, often on the basis of a learning process, without regard to pathophysiologic facts. A disadvantage of neural networks, however, is that unlike the other systems discussed, the "rules" that the network uses do not follow a particular logic and are not explicitly understandable.

GENETIC ALGORITHMS

Genetic algorithms represent another non-knowledge-based method for constructing CDDSS.[28-29] Genetic algorithms take their name from an analogy to the molecular rearrangements that take place in chromosomes. Genes rearrange themselves randomly; such rearrangements give rise to variations in an individual which can affect the individual's ability to pass on genetic material. Over time, the species as a whole incorporates the most adaptive features of the "fittest" individuals. Genetic algorithms take a similar approach. To use a genetic algorithm, the problem to be solved must have many components (e.g., a complex cancer treatment protocol with multiple drugs, radiation therapy, etc.). By selecting components randomly, a population of possible solutions is created. The fittest of these solutions (the one with the best outcome) is selected, and this sub-population undergoes rearrangement, producing another generation of solutions.

By iteratively extracting the best solutions, an optimal solution can be reached. The main challenge in using genetic algorithms is in creating the criteria by which fitness is defined. Since the computing power required to use both genetic algorithms and neural networks is considerable, these techniques have had only limited use in medicine.

SUMMARY

Understanding clinical diagnostic decision support systems (CDDSS) requires a basic understanding of probability and logic. Set theory, familiar to most practitioners who have manipulated collections of literature citations in MEDLINE, provides the basis for understanding probability and other computational methods for reasoning. Probability—in particular, conditional probability—is the principle behind most modern CDDSS, but nonprobabilistic heuristic techniques have been used to good effect in the past. Understanding CDDSS can be facilitated by considering four basic components of the CDDSS process: input, reasoning engine, knowledge base, and output. Input is often constrained by controlled vocabularies or limitations in temporal expression of clinical features. Reasoning engines take on different designs, but their operation is usually transparent to the user of a CDDSS. Knowledge bases contain data from which the reasoning engine takes rules, probabilities, and other constructs required to convert the input into output. Output can take many forms, including a differential diagnosis list or simply a probability of a particular diagnosis. Non-knowledge-based systems use techniques of machine learning to generate methods of turning input into meaningful output, regardless of an explicit representation of expert knowledge.

REFERENCES
1. Behrman RE, Kliegman RM, Arvin AM, eds. Nelson Textbook of Pediatrics, 15th ed. Philadelphia: W.B. Saunders Company, 1996.
2. Shiomi S, Kuroki T, Jomura H et al. Diagnosis of chronic liver disease from liver scintiscans by fuzzy reasoning. J Nuclear Med 1995; 36:593-598.
3. Suryanarayanan S, Reddy NP, Canilang EP. A fuzzy logic diagnosis system for classification of pharyngeal dysphagia. Int J Biomed Comput 1995; 38:207-215.
4. Shortliffe EH. Computer-Based Medical Consultations: MYCIN. New York, NY: Elsevier Computer Science Library, Artificial Intelligence Series, 1976.

5. Kahn MG, Steib SA, Fraser VJ et al. An expert system for culture-based infection control surveillance. Proc Annu Symp Comput Appl Med Care 1993:171-175.
6. Emori TG, Culver DH, Horan TC et al. National Nosocomial Infections Surveillance System (NNIS): description of surveillance methodology. Am J Infect Control 1991; 19:19-35.
7. Bayes T. An essay towards solving a problem in the doctrine of chances. Philosophical Transactions 1763; 3:370-418.
8. Warner HR, Toronto AF, Veasey LG et al. Mathematical approach to medical diagnosis. JAMA 1961; 177:75-81.
9. Warner HR Jr. Iliad: moving medical decision-making into new frontiers. Methods Inf Med 1989; 28:370-372.
10. Shortliffe EH, Buchanan BG. A model of inexact reasoning in medicine. Math Biosci 1975; 23:351-379.
11. Miller R, Masarie FE, Myers J. Quick Medical Reference (QMR) for diagnostic assistance. MD Comput 1986; 3:34-48.
12. Barnett GO, Cimino JJ, Hupp JA et al. DXplain—an evolving diagnostic decision-support system. JAMA 1987; 258:67-74.
13. Tversky A, Kahneman D. Judgment under uncertainty: heuristics and biases. Science 1974; 188:1124-1131.
14. Dawes RM, Faust D, Meehl PE. Clinical versus actuarial judgment. Science 1989; 243:1668-1674.
15. Gigerenzer G, Hoffrage U. How to improve Bayesian reasoning without instruction: frequency formats. Psychol Rev 1995; 102:684-704.
16. Forsythe DE, Buchanan BG, Osheroff JA et al. Expanding the concept of medical information: an observational study of physicians' information needs. Comput Biomed Res 1992; 25:181-200.
17. Aliferis CF, Cooper GF, Miller RA et al. A temporal analysis of QMR. JAMIA 1996; 3:79-91.
18. Kahn CE, Roberts LM, Wang K et al. Preliminary investigation of a Bayesian network for mammographic diagnosis of breast cancer. Proc Annu Symp Comput Appl Med Care 1995;208-212.
19. Miller PL, Frawley SJ, Sayward FG et al. IMM/Serve: An Internet-Accessible Rule-Based Program for Childhood Immunization. Proc Annu Symp Comput Appl Med Care 1995:208-212.
20. Porter JF, Kingsland LCd, Lindberg DA et al. The AI/RHEUM knowledge-based computer consultant system in rheumatology. Performance in the diagnosis of 59 connective tissue disease patients from Japan. Arthritis Rheum 1988; 31:219-226.
21. Tu SW, Eriksson H, Gennari JH et al. Ontology-based configuration of problem-solving methods and generation of knowledge-acquisition tools: application of PROTEGE-II to protocol-based decision support. Artif Intell Med 1995; 7:257-289.
22. Bar-Hillel M. The base-rate fallacy in probability judgments. Acta Psychol 1980; 44:211-233.

23. Musen MA, van der Lei J. Knowledge engineering for clinical consultation programs: modeling the application area. Methods Inf Med 1989; 28:28-35.
24. Mann NH 3d, Brown MD. Artificial intelligence in the diagnosis of low back pain. Orthop Clin North Am 1991; 22:303-314.
25. Wu Y, Giger ML, Doi K et al. Artificial neural networks in mammography: application to decision making in the diagnosis of breast cancer. Radiology 1993; 187:81-87.
26. Astion ML, Wener MH, Thomas RG et al. Application of neural networks to the classification of giant cell arteritis. Arthritis Rheum 1994; 37:760-770.
27. Baxt WG. Use of an artificial neural network for the diagnosis of acute myocardial infarction. Ann Intern Med 1991; 115:843-848.
28. Levin M. Use of genetic algorithms to solve biomedical problems. MD Comput 1995; 12:193-199.
29. Grzymala-Busse JW, Woolery LK. Improving prediction of preterm birth using a new classification scheme and rule induction. Proc Annu Symp Comput Appl Med Care 1994:730-734.

CHAPTER 3

Testing System Accuracy*

Eta S. Berner

Evaluation is a crucial component in the development of any clinical diagnostic decision support system (CDDSS). Much of it takes place informally as part of the development process and is used by the CDDSS developers for system improvement. Once a system is sufficiently mature, more formal evaluation studies should be done, initially of system accuracy and later, of system impact. A wide range of study design choices can be appropriate for assessing accuracy, but once the CDDSS appears to be ready for use in practice, there is a need for more rigorous evaluation. Most published evaluation studies have focused on the issue of system accuracy, with few studies evaluating the impact of using a CDDSS on clinical care. This chapter will address issues involved in assessing the accuracy of CDDSS. Key results from research or evaluation studies of system accuracy will be summarized and discussed. The reader who is interested in the details of individual studies should read the references at the end of this chapter.

As discussed by Miller and Geissbuhler in chapter 1, there are many types of CDDSS. Some are targeted to highly specific problems, such as the those for determining acid-base imbalances,[1] or those

---

Portions of this chapter have been taken verbatim, with permission of the Journal of the Irish Colleges of Physicians and Surgeons, which owns the copyrights, from: Berner, ES. Computer-assisted diagnosis—consensus and controversies. JICPS 1996; 25:43-47.

related to diagnoses in specific organ systems, like the electrocardiographic interpretation programs.[2] The electrocardiographic interpretation (ECG) programs, after years of extensive evaluation, are now routinely in use. Other targeted programs, such as programs to evaluate the acute abdomen, have also had extensive evaluation, although they have not seen as widespread use as the ECG programs.[3-6]

The knowledge-based systems covering a broad domain of complaints and diseases, that will be the focus of this chapter, have become increasingly visible in recent years. Examples of programs which are commercially available include DXplain, Iliad, Meditel, Problem-Knowledge Coupler and QMR.[7-11] All of these programs have menu-driven data entry, and all generate a list of possible diagnoses to explain the patient's findings. In some of the programs, text describing specific associations of symptoms and diseases, references, or other information can be viewed by the user; in others, the program only produces the list of diagnostic hypotheses. The programs vary in the specific diseases included in their knowledge base, the type of information they can accept, the particular algorithms they use, the user interface, the way the data are displayed, and in the opportunity for user interaction with the program. In general, these programs have only limited ability to accept descriptions of the duration and sequence of symptoms. This chapter will summarize results of published research studies on the accuracy of CDDSS and highlight those areas where controversy still exists.

PERFORMANCE OF CDDSS

Studies testing the accuracy of CDDSS have used a variety of types of cases, including simulated cases, real inpatient and outpatient cases, and extremely difficult cases, such as CPC cases published in the *New England Journal of Medicine*. In general, the research paradigm has involved input of patient case data into the CDDSS and judgments of the appropriateness of the diagnostic suggestions produced by the system after it analyzed the case data. In some studies, expert users entered the case data into the system, in others, nonexperts. While some researchers only evaluated the accuracy of the top diagnosis suggested by the CDDSS, others examined all of the diagnoses produced for a given case and judged their accuracy. Given the differences in the CDDSS themselves and these differences in study design, it is not surprising that CDDSS show varying performance data. While there is a wide range of performance, the data from these different studies do show that CDDSS performance, while far from perfect, is better than might be expected, especially since many of the systems were tested on particularly challenging cases. Also, in the few studies which tested different CDDSS on the same set of clinical case data, the performances of the different CDDSS were surprisingly similar. Overall, the research results show that these systems are capable of suggesting the correct diagnosis for a particular case as a possibility at least half the time, and possibly close to 90% of the time, if the patient's diagnosis is in the system's knowledge base.[9,12-37]

Part of the variation in accuracy estimates can be attributed to genuine performance differences among the CDDSS. Other differences are due to the variations in study design described above. In most studies that used real patient cases, the specific diagnosis for a given case was determined by a definitive laboratory test, a biopsy or autopsy results. If simulated cases were used, or if there is no definitive test for the particular diagnosis, expert consensus might be used to determine the correct case diagnosis. There were also variations in the conditions under which the CDDSS were evaluated, e.g., the test cases were, or were not, all in the systems' knowledge base. While the variations in study design can be discerned fairly readily from the published articles, the impact of these differences in understanding CDDSS performance is unclear. In addition to these differences in study design, there is a more subtle reason for the differences in performance results.

Miller and Geissbuhler note, in the first chapter of this book, that there are different conceptions of what constitutes the diagnostic process. What is not generally appreciated is that researchers trying to determine whether the computer's suggestions are "correct" often use different definitions of what they mean by the "correct" diagnosis. To illustrate this point, virtually anyone would agree that the computer's suggestion was correct if it produced the definitive final diagnosis (e.g., Kreutzfeld-Jakob disease) or its exact synonym (subacute spongiform encephalopathy). There may be more disagreement as to whether the computer is correct if it produces something very close to the exact diagnosis, perhaps the broader class into which the specific diagnosis fell, such as viral encephalopathy. However, if a CDDSS suggests something even farther from the specific diagnosis, that is so general that it hardly helps to narrow the possibilities, determination of whether that diagnosis is correct becomes even more problematic. For instance, in one study, the author, who also developed the CDDSS, counted a computer diagnosis of "carcinoma" as correct for a patient whose actual definitive diagnosis was a malignant colon polyp and whose initial findings were fatigue and anemia.[36] Other judges might consider such a general description as "carcinoma" too imprecise to be labeled as the correct diagnosis. Differences in the criteria may affect some systems more than others, since decision support systems vary in the specificity and granularity of their terminology. That is, if the CDDSS developer knows that carcinoma is as specific as his system can be because its controlled vocabulary does not include any specific cancers, the developer might consider the general diagnosis correct, whereas an expert panel in a research study or a clinician using the system who may be unfamiliar with the details of the system vocabulary might not be so generous.

It is generally assumed that the CDDSS needs to be accurate so that it can be of assistance to the clinician who is seeking its advice and so the patient will not be harmed by inappropriate or costly work-up or treatment. An issue related to the question of precision of diagnostic suggestions is whether a CDDSS can give an incorrect diagnosis and still be helpful. Although at first glance this may seem counterintuitive, there are several ways that such a situation could arise. A CDDSS could suggest a specific diagnosis, such as histoplasmosis, when the patient actually had a different fungal infection.[24] It is possible that the physician, who might not have been thinking of fungal infections at all, could more readily arrive at the correct diagnosis than she would have without the suggestion from the CDDSS. At the more extreme end of the continuum, even if the CDDSS suggests a completely wrong diagnosis, if the work-up or treatment would be the same as that for the correct diagnosis, there may be no difference in the outcome for the patient and by leading the clinician to the correct diagnosis might actually improve patient care.

These differences among systems and criteria for determining accuracy make it difficult to compare the results of different studies, even with similar research designs, since the decision making criteria as to accuracy standards are often not explicit and rarely appear in published articles. They also underscore that while accuracy of the system per se is important, the "bottom line" should still be the impact of the CDDSS on the clinician's decision making.

While the percentage of correct diagnoses varies among studies, in almost all of the studies, the correct diagnosis is rarely the only diagnosis suggested by the CDDSS. All of the CDDSS generate other diagnoses that the system considers as possibilities, but many of these, in some cases over half of the total suggested, are ones that a medically knowledgeable user might easily be able to exclude as not relevant to the particular case. It is not clear whether the high percentage of irrelevant diagnoses is a result of the physician's knowing more about the patient than can be entered into the CDDSS, or because of limitations in the programs' reasoning algorithms. Even for the systems which tend to produce more focused lists of suggestions when analyzing diseases in their knowledge base, there is still a good deal of "noise" that must be distinguished from "signal."

Even if one errs on the side of caution in accepting the results of these studies, it is probably safe to say that in at least half of the cases, most of the CDDSS that have been studied are likely to suggest diagnoses that most observers would consider specific enough to be potentially helpful to the user. We also know that these relevant diagnoses may sometimes be buried in a list of nonrelevant diagnostic suggestions.

Although the research data are fairly consistent on the level of functioning of these programs, there is lack of agreement on how to interpret what the data mean and on other issues related to their use. Some areas of controversy include: (1) how to interpret the performance data; (2) who should be the primary users of the systems; (3) the types of cases for which the programs should be used; and (4) the methods by which these systems should be evaluated. In addition, since many of the CDDSS can be used in other ways than simply suggesting diagnoses, there is controversy about which CDDSS functions should be evaluated.

INTERPRETATION OF PERFORMANCE DATA

Schoolman[38] has suggested that performance data on these systems, e.g., sensitivity and specificity, be provided so that users can judge their accuracy. However, the same performance data can lead to different conclusions. When a software reviewer writes in a journal that a given program performed well or poorly, the review is often followed by letters from users who perceive the system differently.[39-40] Since software reviews generally are based on small samples of cases, one reason for these differing opinions may be differential performance across cases.[41] Another reason may be that different individuals vary in their tolerance for the irrelevant information that is produced. It is also probable that program performance is related to the proficiency of the users with the particular software. However, even when several systems are evaluated on the same sample of cases and the performance criteria are carefully described,[31] there are still differences of opinion as to the implications of the data. In an accompanying editorial to the article by Berner et al.,[31] the editor gave the programs a grade of "C."[42] A subsequent letter to the editor said the grade should at least be a "B."[43] Clearly there are reasons for different interpretations of the data that may not be solved by even very systematic studies of performance.

Performance Standards

One problem involves difficulty in determining the standard to which the programs should be compared. A simplistic answer is that what we expect of the programs is that they should perform like an ideal diagnostic consultant, which would mean virtually always considering the correct diagnosis and only suggesting plausible diagnoses to rule out. While this may be the ideal standard, there is evidence that expert diagnosticians are farther from perfect than we would like to think, and that there is more disagreement among experts than might be expected.[44-46] In fact, the data from the studies by Elstein, Murphy and their colleagues[34-35] on the impact of CDDSS on physician diagnoses showed that without using the CDDSS, University faculty physicians considered the correct diagnosis within their top six diagnoses only half the time, and residents and students performed even worse. Perhaps a standard of "better performance than the average clinician" would be appropriate, but such data are almost impossible to obtain reliably.

It is also likely that individuals have different opinions as to the importance of the various performance measures. The CDDSS generally provides a list of possible diagnoses, rather than a single right answer. Some clinicians undoubtedly prefer a lengthy list of diagnostic possibilities and will tolerate the extra diagnoses that they can ignore. For these users, failure to include the diagnosis that the patient actually has might be more of a problem than lack of specificity. Other clinicians demand a list that includes the correct diagnosis enough times to make it worthwhile for them to use the CDDSS, but one which is focused enough to help them develop a reasonable work-up plan. For these clinicians, long lists of diagnoses that require their attention might be a major drawback.

The interpretation of the performance results is in part dependent on the intended use of the CDDSS. The accuracy standards to which a CDDSS must be held if it is expected to function in place of a physician should be very high. While high standards may be desirable for any use of the CDDSS, they are not absolutely necessary if one assumes that a knowledgeable professional will filter the system's suggestions, using what is helpful and discarding what is not helpful. Although some individuals have suggested that decision support systems might eventually replace the physician as a diagnostician,[47-48] most developers of these programs emphasize that they are not designed for such a purpose.[49-50] Given that (1) the CDDSS developers never intended them to replace the physician; (2) the current systems cannot incorporate all of the information about patients that physicians use in their own diagnostic thinking and (3) many of the knowledge bases may be incomplete even with further expansion over their current status, even if their performance improved significantly, CDDSS are most likely to remain a support tool that prompts the physician's thinking, rather a substitute for the physician's judgment

Appropriate Cases

Another important issue is the identification of situations or types of cases for which these programs can be optimally used. Because the currently available CDDSS for the most part require separate data entry from the information entered into the patient's medical record, time constraints may prevent their routine use. However, as technology improves and automated data entry into these programs becomes feasible, an important unresolved issue is whether they should be used for every patient. Miller[12] has suggested that one of the paradoxes of broad-based CDDSS is that the puzzling cases for which the systems are appropriate, and on which most of the performance testing has focused, may not occur often enough to warrant frequent use of the systems. It is not known whether performance on difficult cases generalizes to use with the more routine problems that make up the large proportion of physicians' practices. Also, even if diagnostic advice were available on all patients, users of the systems would most likely attend to the advice only on the cases where they are uncertain about the diagnosis. Thus, the overconfident physician, who may be most in need of decision support, may be least likely to use these programs. It is also possible that these systems would be most useful to clinicians whose expertise lies outside the domain for which the systems were developed (e.g., an internal medicine system may be more useful to an obstetrician-gynecologist than to an internist), yet specialists may not appreciate the need to seek decision support from a system outside their own specialty.

EXPERTISE OF THE USERS

The developers of most of the broad-based CDDSS expect that medically knowledgeable individuals will use the systems in an appropriate manner. At present, how knowledgeable the user must be is undefined, but given that a great deal of sifting through the program output is necessary, the user must be able to recognize erroneous information. Some people have suggested that "medically knowledgeable" does not necessarily mean that a physician will be the primary user[48] and that medical students, physicians' assistants, or nurses might all be able to use the program appropriately. Weed[10,51-52] has a CDDSS designed for input by a nonphysician, although it is expected that a physician will review the diagnostic suggestions produced. While less experienced clinicians may need more diagnostic assistance than seasoned physicians, the novices may also be less able than experts to evaluate the system's suggestions.

EVALUATION METHODS

There is debate about what constitutes adequate evaluation. There are arguments that the only evaluation studies worth considering are those from well designed clinical trials of the CDDSS in actual use.[53-55] Johnston et al. conducted a literature review of all types of decision support systems and concluded that these systems were of limited use.[54] However, they based their conclusions on only the few studies reviewed that fit their very strict methodological criteria, and most of those reviewed were not the broad-based diagnostic systems. Other researchers have felt that a broader view of acceptable evaluation is warranted, especially in the earlier stages of development.[31,56]

Although evaluation paradigms other than randomized controlled trials can provide valuable information about CDDSS, the question of whether, or when in the developmental process, outside evaluation is necessary is still unresolved. Many studies of a variety of computer-assisted diagnostic programs, not just the broad-based ones, have been conducted by the program developers themselves or individuals closely associated with them.[7,14,16,18,19,21,30,33,57] When outsiders evaluate the same programs, the results are often less positive.[5,6,15,17,31,32,34,35] It is often difficult to tell whether the discrepant results are because of differences in study design as has been suggested,[58] whether the developers use more lenient standards, or whether the programs are not as transferable across settings as might be desired.

In addition to the issue of who should conduct the evaluation, there is a question of what aspects of the CDDSS should be evaluated. Most of the studies examining CDDSS accuracy have focused on the ability of the system to generate a list of diagnostic hypotheses. While this is an important capability for any CDDSS, and the major function for some, it is not the only manner in which many CDDSS can be used. In surveying physicians who had purchased QMR, Berner and Maisiak found that while almost all the physicians felt they were proficient in using the electronic textbook functions that permitted them to view the findings associated with various diseases, only 60% felt comfortable using the case analysis function which has been the primary CDDSS capability evaluated in the literature.[59] Miller has cautioned that the performance of CDDSS may vary depending on which functions are evaluated and that blanket conclusions about the overall accuracy of a CDDSS cannot be made from evaluation of only one aspect.[60] More research is needed on how physicians actually use the programs to determine on which aspects of the CDDSS the evaluation effort should focus.

To date, there has been very little research published on the use of these CDDSS by clinicians who were not involved with the development of the programs, despite the calls for trials of these systems in actual practice.[53-55] Research currently being conducted by Berner and her colleagues and Elstein and his collaborators, while not examining the effects of these systems in actual clinical practice, are using as subjects physicians who were not part of the CDDSS development teams and who have varying familiarity with the programs. While this information will be very useful, the issue of how these systems affect clinical care when used in practice by physicians still needs to be addressed. Thus, there is clear consensus that good research on the use of CDDSS is needed, but there are too few published studies at this time to draw firm conclusions as to the effectiveness of the broad-based CDDSS in clinical practice.

CONCLUSIONS

Good evaluation of these complex diagnostic systems is not an easy task. Anecdotal reviews do not meet appropriate standards of scientific rigor, and large scale comparative studies of program performance such as those done to test electrocardiographic interpretation programs[2] and the research by Berner, Elstein and their colleagues[31,32,34,35] are very time consuming and expensive. Well-controlled trials of use of these systems in clinical practice may be even more costly, since appropriately challenging cases on which to test the broad-based diagnostic systems are, almost by definition, not going to be those that are readily available.

While there may be debate as to the bottom line "grade" for these broad-based computer-assisted diagnostic programs, any grades at this point in their development are really indicators of progress, not a final grade. Most developers, users and evaluators of these programs would agree that there is still a great deal of room for improvement. The programs certainly have potential, but whether it will be realized on a large scale remains to be seen. Computer technology is rapidly advancing and other models of decision support systems are being developed, as discussed in other chapters in this book. Whether the currently available systems become more widely used will depend in part on whether they continue to expand their knowledge bases and begin to explore automated data entry and integration with other computer-based systems, which are part of the normal work-flow of the physician. Both of these developments are starting to occur.[61]

Research is needed to begin to resolve the areas of controversy. Obviously, the ultimate test for these kinds of systems will be clinical trials on the impact of their use in multiple practice settings (see chapter 8). However, we also need to examine how these systems assist users at different levels of medical expertise, discover how easy they are to use in a busy practice situation, and determine the optimal way to integrate computer-assisted diagnostic systems into the practice of medicine so that we can evaluate their effects on patient care.

REFERENCES

1. Bleich HL. Computer evaluation of acid-base disorders. J Clin Invest 1969; 48:1689-1696.
2. Willems JL, Abreu-Lima C, Arnaud P et al. The diagnostic performance of computer programs for the interpretation of electrocardiograms. N Engl J Med 1991; 325:1767-1773.
3. de Dombal, FT. The diagnosis of acute abdominal pain with computer assistance: worldwide perspective. Ann Chir 1991; 45:273-277.
4. Adams ID, Chan M, Clifford PC et al. Computer aided diagnosis of acute abdominal pain: a multicentre study. Br Med J (Clin Res Ed) 1986; 293:800-804.
5. Sutton GC. How accurate is computer-aided diagnosis? Lancet 1989; 2:905-908.
6. Gough IR. Computer assisted diagnosis of the acute abdomen. Aust N Z J Surg 1993; 63:699-702.
7. Barnett GO, Cimino JJ, Hupp JA et al. DXplain—an evolving diagnostic decision-support system. JAMA 1987; 258:67-74.
8. Warner HR Jr. Iliad: moving medical decision-making into new frontiers. Methods Inf Med 1989; 28:370-372.
9. Waxman HS, Worley WE. Computer-assisted adult medical diagnosis: subject review and evaluation of a new microcomputer-based system. Medicine 1990; 69:125-136.
10. Weed LL. Knowledge Coupling: New Premises and New Tools for Medical Care and Education. New York, NY: Springer-Verlag, 1991.
11. Miller R, Masarie FE, Myers J. Quick Medical Reference (QMR) for diagnostic assistance. MD Comput 1986; 3:34-48.
12. Miller RA. Medical diagnostic decision support systems—past, present, and future: a threaded bibliography and commentary. JAMIA 1994; 1:8-27.
13. Georgakis DC, Trace DA, Naeymi-Rad F et al. A statistical evaluation of the diagnostic performance of MEDAS—the medical emergency decision assistance system. Proc Annu Symp Comput Appl Med Care 1990:815-819.
14. Nelson SJ, Blois MS, Tuttle MS et al. Evaluating RECONSIDER: a computer program for diagnostic prompting. J Med Sys 1985; 9:379-388.
15. Hammersley JR, Cooney K. Evaluating the utility of available differential diagnosis systems. Proc Annu Symp Comput Appl Med Care 1988:229-231.
16. Feldman MJ, Barnett GO. An approach to evaluating the accuracy of DXplain. Comput Methods Programs Biomed 1991; 35:261-266.
17. Heckerling PS, Elstein AS, Terzian CG et al. The effect of incomplete knowledge on the diagnosis of a computer consultant system. Med Inf 1991; 16:363-370.
18. Lau LM, Warner HR. Performance of a diagnostic system (Iliad) as a tool for quality assurance. Comput Biomed Res 1992; 25:314-323.

19. Barness LA, Tunnessen WW Jr, Worley WE et al. Computer-assisted diagnosis in pediatrics. Am J Dis Child 1974; 127:852-858.
20. O'Shea JS. Computer-assisted pediatric diagnosis. Am J Dis Child 1975; 129:199-202.
21. Swender PT, Tunnessen WW Jr, Oski FA. Computer-assisted diagnosis. Am J Dis Child 1974; 127:859-861.
22. Wexler JR, Swender PT, Tunnessen WW Jr et al. Impact of a system of computer-assisted diagnosis. Initial evaluation of the hospitalized patient. Am J Dis Child 1975; 129:203-205.
23. Bankowitz RA, Lave JR, McNeil MA. A method for assessing the impact of a computer-based decision support system on health care outcomes. Methods Inf Med 1992; 31:3-11.
24. Bankowitz RA, McNeil MA, Challinor SM et al. A computer-assisted medical diagnostic consultation service: implementation and prospective evaluation of a prototype. Ann Intern Med 1989; 110:824-832.
25. Bankowitz RA, McNeil MA, Challinor SM et al. Effect of a computer-assisted general medicine diagnostic consultation service on housestaff diagnostic strategy. Methods Inf Med 1989; 28:352-356.
26. Berman L, Miller RA. Problem area formation as an element of computer aided diagnosis: a comparison of two strategies within quick medical reference (QMR). Methods Inf Med 1991; 30:90-95.
27. Middleton B, Shwe MA, Heckerman DE et al. Probabilistic diagnosis using a reformulation of the Internist-1/QMR knowledge base. II. Evaluation of diagnostic performance. Methods Inf Med 1991; 30:256-267.
28. Miller RA, Pople HE Jr, Myers J. Internist-I, an experimental computer-based diagnostic consultant for general internal medicine. N Engl J Med 1982; 307:468-476.
29. Miller RA, Masarie FE Jr. The quick medical reference (QMR) relationships function: description and evaluation of a simple, efficient "multiple diagnoses" algorithm. Medinfo 1992:512-518.
30. Miller RA, McNeil MA, Challinor S et al. Status Report: The Internist-1 / Quick Medical Reference project. West J Med 1986; 145:816-822.
31. Berner ES, Webster GD, Shugerman AA et al. Performance of four computer-based diagnostic systems. N Engl J Med 1994; 330:1792-1796.
32. Berner ES, Jackson JR, Algina J. Relationships among performance scores of four diagnostic decision support systems. JAMIA 1996; 3:208-215.
33. Bankowitz, RA. The effectiveness of QMR in medical decision support. Executive summary and final report. Springfield, VA: U.S. Department of Commerce, National Technical Information Service, 1994.
34. Murphy GC, Friedman CP, Elstein AS. The influence of a decision support system on the differential diagnosis of medical practitioners

at three levels of training. Proc AMIA Fall Symp Comput 1996:
219-223.

35. Elstein AS, Friedman CP, Wolf FM et al. Effects of a decision support system on the diagnostic accuracy of users: a preliminary report. JAMIA 1996; 3:422-428.

36. Innis MD. Medisets. Computer-assisted diagnosis using a modified
set theory. Proc Second Natl Health Conf, Health Informatics Conf,
'94, Gold Coast Australia, 1994, 286-291.

37. Bacchus CM, Quinton C, O'Rourke K et al. A ramdomized crossover trial of quick medical reference (QMR) as a teaching tool for
medical interns. J Gen Intern Med 1994; 9:616-621.

38. Schoolman HM. Obligations of the expert system builder: meeting
the needs of the user. MD Comput 1991; 8:316-321.

39. Diamond I.W. A different view of ILIAD. MD Comput 1992; 9:76-77.

40. Waxman HS, Worley WE. Computer-assisted diagnosis. Ann Intern
Med 1990; 113:561.

41. Berner ES. The problem with software reviews of decision support
systems. MD Comput 1993; 10:8-12.

42. Kassirer JP. A report card on computer-assisted diagnosis—the grade:
C. N Engl J Med 1994; 330:1824-1825.

43. de Dombal FT. Computer-assisted diagnosis in Europe. N Engl J Med
1994; 331:1238.

44. Anderson RE, Hill RB, Key CR. The sensitivity and specificity of clinical diagnostics during five decades. JAMA 1989; 261.1610-1617.

45. Chimowitz MI, Logigian EL, Caplan LR. The accuracy of bedside
neurological diagnoses. Ann Neurol 1990; 28:78-87,

46. Elmore JG, Wells CK, Lee CH et al. Variability in radiologists' interpretation of mammograms. N Engl J Med 1994; 331:1493-1499.

47. Mazoue JG. Diagnosis without doctors. J Med Philos 1990; 15:
559-579.

48. Yolton RL. Computer-based diagnostic systems. N Engl J Med 1994;
331:1023.

49. Miller RA, Masarie FE Jr. The demise of the "Greek Oracle" model
for medical diagnosis systems. Methods Inf Med 1990; 29:1-2.

50. Miller RA. Why the standard view is standard: people, not machines,
understand patients' problems. J Med Philos 1990; 15:581-591.

51. Weed LL. Problem-knowledge couplers: Philosophy, use and interpretation. PKC Corporation 1982; pgs. 2-22.

52. Weed LL. Reengineering medicine: questions and answers. Federation Bull 1995; 82:24-36.

53. Heathfield HA, Wyatt J. Philosophies for the design and development of clinical decision-support systems. Methods Inf Med 1993;
32:1-8.

54. Johnston ME, Langton KB, Haynes RB et al. Effects of computer-
based clinical decision support systems on clinician performance and

patient outcome:a critical appraisal of research. Ann Intern Med 1994; 120:135-142.
55. Wyatt J, Spiegelhalter D. Field trials of medical decision-aids: potential problems and solutions. Proc Annu Symp Comput Appl Med Care 1991:3-7.
56. Miller PL. The evaluation of artificial intelligence systems in medicine. Comput Methods Programs Biomed 1986; 22:5-11.
57. McAdam WA, Brock BM, Armitage T et al. Twelve years experience of computer-aided diagnosis in a district general hospital. Ann R Coll Surg Engl 1990; 72:140-146.
58. de Dombal FT. Computer-aided decision support:in praise of level playing fields. Methods Inf Med 1994; 33:161-163.
59. Berner ES, Maisiak RS. Physician use of interactive functions in diagnostic decision support systems. Proc AMIA Fall Symp 1997; 842.
60. Miller RA. Evaluating evaluations of medical diagnostic systems. JAMIA 1996; 3:429-431.
61. Welford CR. A comprehensive computerized patient record with automated linkage to QMR. Proc Annu Symp Comput Appl Med Care 1994: 814-818.

Part II

Applications of
Clinical Diagnostic
Decision Support Systems

CHAPTER 4

Hospital-Based Decision Support

Peter J. Haug, Reed M. Gardner and R. Scott Evans

Decision support technologies are becoming increasingly available to medical practitioners. In recent years, a variety of programs designed to assist with drug dosing, health maintenance, diagnosis and other clinically relevant decisions have been developed for the medical market. Increasing ease of access to personal computers is partially responsible for this growth. So is the interest in automated medical decision-making that has grown from an expanding awareness of the successes of medical computing.

Much of the literature that has sparked this awareness comes from research done on an older generation of medical information systems. These systems reside on large mainframe computing hardware. Many of them have served hospitals and have supported the patient care given there.[1,2] The applications and algorithms that were piloted in these systems have provided the background for the modern decision support technologies which we see developing and evolving in client/server environments and on personal computers.

Contributors to the body of knowledge of applying computer systems to clinical practice include the several sites where hospital-based, medical decision support have been implemented and studied. Among the leaders in these efforts have been groups at the Regenstrief Institute in Indianapolis,[3] Columbia Presbyterian Medical Center in New York,[4] and Beth Israel Hospital in Boston.[5] Recent efforts to incorporate decision support into order entry systems at the Brigham and Women's Hospital in Boston[6] and Vanderbilt University Medical Center in Nashville[7] are helping to define the direction that hospital-based computing will follow in the future.

In this chapter, we will discuss medical decision support applications that help provide clinical care in a hospital setting. The principal source of the examples come from the HELP Hospital Information System (HIS) located at the LDS Hospital in Salt Lake City and developed by the members of the Department of Medical Informatics of the University of Utah.[8] As a part of our description of decision support applications in the HELP system, we will discuss the data used and the mechanism through which suggested decisions are communicated to the user. In addition we will review a set of applications, developed and tested within the HELP system, that include an element of "diagnostic" decision support.

Truly "diagnostic" systems have been a perpetual theme in medical informatics research. However, systems featuring a diagnostic paradigm are rarely found in routine hospital clinic services. More common are systems that depend on simple algorithms to inform and remind users of important clinical data or of medical facts which may change decisions they have made, or will make. Examples of these include decision support tools that critique medication orders and the system for identifying life-threatening laboratory results which are described below.

The HELP system includes two types of clinical diagnostic decision support systems (CDDSS). The first type focuses on narrowly circumscribed medical conditions; these systems are in daily clinical use. The systems include those that recognize clinical syndromes such as adverse drug events or those that attempt to determine from microbiology data and other information which pathogens are important causes of infection. The second type of diagnostic systems are those that attempt to discriminate among a group of important diagnostic entities using raw medical data. These diagnostic systems often attempt the challenging task of managing large degrees of uncertainty using pattern matching algorithms. Several of these types of systems have been, or are being, tested in the HELP environment. Below we describe experience with three of these more aggressive diagnostic programs.

THE HELP SYSTEM

The overall setting for much of the work described here is the HELP Hospital Information System (HIS) operating in the LDS Hospital. HELP stands for Health Evaluation through Logical Processes and is a culmination of more than 20 years of development and testing.[8] It currently operates on high availability hardware supplied by the Tandem Computer Corporation. Recently, principal software components of the HELP system have also been installed in seven of the hospitals operated by Intermountain Health Care (IHC). At the LDS Hospital, the information system communicates with users and developers through approximately 1,250 terminals and more than 200 printers. The system is interfaced to a variety of other computer systems including a billing system, a laboratory system, an electrocardiography system, a medical records system, a digital radiology system, and a collection of local area networks (LANs) used by a variety of departments for local research and departmental management functions.

The HELP System consists of an integrated clinical database, a frame-based medical decision-support system, programs to support hospital and departmental administrative functions, and the software tools needed to maintain and expand these components. The integrated clinical database contains a variety of patient data kept online during the patient's stay. This database can be accessed by health care professionals at terminals throughout the hospital. Terminals allow the entry of pertinent clinical data into the HELP system by all personnel who are involved in patient care. Table 4.1 is a partial list of the data in the system.

Use of the HELP system for decision support has been a major focus of research since the system's inception. The result has been a set of embedded expert system development tools. The HELP System contains a decision support subsystem based on a modular representation of medical decision logic in frames.[9] This set of tools has led to the successful development of expert systems in blood gas interpretation,[10] intensive care settings,[11] and medication monitoring,[12] to name a few. The syntax used in the decision system is currently being extended to allow use of Arden Syntax, an American Society for Testing and Materials (ASTM) standard for medical decision logic.[13] The HELP System hardware and software environment has provided the setting for the implementation and testing of the decision support tools described below.

Table 4.1. Partial list of data in HELP system

Clinical Data Routinely Captured by the HELP Hospital Information System

Chemistry	Hematology
Medications	X-ray Findings
Allergies	Dietary Information
Blood Gases	Surgical Procedures
Electrocardiograms	ICU Monitoring
Intake/Output	Pulmonary Function
Demographic Information	Microbiology
Cardiac Catheterization Data	Respiratory Therapy Notes
Biopsy Results	Nursing Data
Select Physical Examination	Pathology Department Data
Admit/Discharge Information	History and Physical Exam Reports
Consult Reports	Procedure Reports

CATEGORIES OF DECISION SUPPORT TECHNOLOGIES

Independent of the environment in which they are used, two elements of medical decision support applications are critical to their success. These are: (1) the mechanism by which the systems acquire the data used in their decision algorithms; and (2) the interface through which they interact with clinicians to report their results. These considerations have led us to describe different categorizations of decision support.[14] Although somewhat arbitrary, this categorization captures the idea that different models of computerized assistance may be needed for different types of clinical problems.

The four categories are: (1) processes which respond to clinical data by issuing an alert; (2) programs that respond to recorded decisions to alter care (typically new orders) by critiquing the decision and proposing alternative suggestions as appropriate; (3) applications that respond to a request by the decision maker by suggesting a set of diagnostic or therapeutic maneuvers fitted to the patient's needs; and (4) retrospective quality assurance applications where clinical data are abstracted from patient records and decisions about the quality of care are made and fed back to caregivers. We will describe the first three types in this chapter.

ALERTING SYSTEMS

Alerting processes are programs that function continuously, monitoring select clinical data as it is stored in the patient's electronic record. They are designed to test specific types of data against pre-defined criteria. If the data meet the criteria these systems alert medical personnel. The timing and character of the messages vary with the alerting goals.

A typical example is a subsystem implemented on the HELP system which monitors common laboratory results and detects and alerts for potentially life-threatening abnormalities in the data acquired. This application is notable for the simplicity of its decision logic, as well as for the magnitude of its potential impact.

The HELP system captures results from the clinical laboratory through an interface to a dedicated laboratory information system (LIS). The results are collected and returned to the HELP system for storage in the clinical record as soon as they are collected and validated in the LIS.

Laboratory results are reviewed by personnel engaged in patient care both through terminals connected to the HELP system and through a variety of special and general-purpose printouts, such as rounds reports generated by the HELP system. The "times" when the data are reviewed have only a loose relationship to the "times" when they become available. Instead, the principal review time determinant is typically the work schedules of the physicians and nurses involved with the patient. The physician, for instance, may visit the hospital twice a day for rounds and review patient data only during those times unless some aspect of the patient's condition prompts a more aggressive approach.

Under these circumstances, abnormalities in laboratory results, especially those that are unexpected, may not receive the timely attention they deserve. In particular, unexpected laboratory abnormalities may go unseen for hours until a nurse or physician reviews them during their routine activities. Or, as some authors have noted, they may be missed entirely.[15-16]

As a response to this disparity, Karen Bradshaw/Tate and her associates have described an experiment with a Computerized Laboratory Alerting System (CLAS) designed to bring potentially life-threatening conditions to the attention of care givers.[17-20] This system was constructed by reducing a set of 60 alerts developed during a previous pilot system development[21] to the 10 most important conditions (Table 4.2).

Six medical experts from the disciplines of surgery, cardiology, internal medicine, and critical care participated in the development of these alerts and the system used to deliver them. The alerts chosen were translated into computer logic and tested to determine that the logic functioned properly. Data from previously admitted patients were used to refine the logic.

Once the logic was deemed acceptable, an experiment was designed to evaluate the effect of the system on several intermediate outcome measures. Two approaches were tested for delivering the alerts. The first of these techniques was tested on a single nursing division to determine its acceptability. A flashing yellow light was installed in the division and whenever an alert was generated for a patient in that division the light was activated. It continued to flash until the alert was reviewed and acknowledged on a computer terminal. The second approach was less intrusive to the nursing staff. Whenever anyone entered the program used to review a patient's laboratory results, any unacknowledged alerts for that patient were immediately displayed along with the data that had triggered them.

The results of this type of intervention were tested in three ways. First, appropriateness of treatment was evaluated. The alerting system was shown to result in significantly more appropriate therapy for conditions involving abnormalities of Na^+, K^+ and glucose. Second, time spent in the life-threatening condition with and without the alerting system was examined. The length of time in the life-threatening condition dropped in each of the alerting subgroups analyzed. Finally, the hospital length of stay was examined. A significant improvement in this parameter was also noted for the patients with abnormalities of Na^+, K^+ or glucose.

This type of decision support intervention is becoming increasingly common as hospital information systems evolve.[22] In the inpatient environment, where the severity of illness is steadily increasing, there is a strong potential for better alerting systems to improve quality of patient care.

Table 4.2. Alerts for which computerized alerting logic was created

Alerting Condition	Criteria
Hyponatremia (NAL)	$Na^+ < 120$ mEq/l
Falling Sodium (NAF) mEq/l	Na^+ fallen 15+ mEq/l in 24 hr. and $Na^+ < 130$
Hypernatremia (NAH)	$Na^+ > 155$ mEq/l
Hypokalemia (KL)	$K^+ < 2.7$ mEq/l
Falling Potassium (KLF)	K^+ fallen 1+ mEq/l in 24 hr. and $K^+ < 3.2$ mEq/l
Hypokalemia, patient on digoxin (KLD)	$K^+ < 3.3$ mEq/l and patient on digoxin
Hyperkalemia (KH)	$K^+ > 6.0$ mEq/l
Metabolic acidosis (CO_2L)	$CO_2 < 15$ and BUN > 50 or $CO_2 < 18$ and BUN < 50 or $CO_2 < 18$ (BUN unknown) or CO_2 fallen 10+ in 24 hr and $CO_2 < 25$
Hypoglycemia (GL)	Glucose < 45 mg%
Hyperglycemia (GH)	Glucose > 500 mg%

CRITIQUING SYSTEMS

In the alerting example described above, the computer system responded to elements in the data base by prompting those caring for the patient to intervene. In contrast, critiquing processes begin functioning when an order for a medical intervention is entered into the information system. Such methods typically respond by evaluating an order and either pointing out disparities between the order and an internal definition of proper care or by proposing an alternative therapeutic approach. Below we describe a critiquing subsystem that specifically targets orders for blood products.

In recent years it has become increasingly apparent that, while the transfusion of blood products is an important, often life-saving therapy, these same blood products must be ordered and administered with care. Not only are there significant reasons for anxiety concerning diseases that can be transmitted during transfusions, but, in addition, the limited supply and short shelf life of blood products make them a scarce resource to be used sparingly. In 1987 the Joint Commission for the Accreditation of Healthcare Organizations (JCAHO) released a document outlining nine steps to be taken in the review of institutional blood usage.[23] Central to this document was a requirement for health care institutions to develop criteria for the use of blood products and to carefully monitor compliance with these criteria.

At the LDS Hospital the response to these requirements was to develop a computer system designed specifically to manage the ordering of blood transfusions and to assist in ensuring compliance with criteria for proper use of blood products.[24-26] A central premise of the system design was that all orders would be entered into the computer and that physicians or nurses would enter all blood orders.

Embedded into the blood-ordering program is a critiquing tool designed to ascertain the reason for every transfusion and to compare the reason to strict criteria specific to the type of transfusion planned. For instance, when an order is made for packed red blood cells, the criteria in Table 4.3 below are used to critique the order.

The process of entering an order into this system includes several points at which information bearing on the propriety of giving blood products is displayed. As a first step, the physician is shown the blood products ordered in the last 24 hours. This is followed by a display of the applicable laboratory data. Then the user chooses the specific blood products required along with the number of units and the priority (stat, routine, etc.). At this point the user is asked to document the reason for the order. A list of reasons, specific to the blood product chosen, is displayed and the user chooses the appropriate rationale for the intervention. The computer then applies the stored criteria and determines whether the order meets the hospital's guidelines.

If the guidelines are met, the order is logged and the blood bank and nursing division are informed electronically and via computer printout. If the criteria are not met, the user is presented with a message stating the applicable criteria and relevant patient data. The physician or nurse may optionally decide to place or cancel the order, but he or she is required to enter (as free text) the reasons for the decision to override the system.

The criteria used are the result of an effort by the LDS Hospital medical staff. The criteria were developed primarily by using published guidelines, but with some adaptations for local conditions (altitude of 4,500 feet). The criteria have undergone several modifications based on experience as well as new definitions of standards for these therapies.

Table 4.3. Simplified criteria for ordering packed red blood cells

Hemoglobin < 12 g/dl or hematocrit < 35% if age ≥ 35 years
Hemoglobin < 10 g/dl or hematocrit < 30% if age < 35 years
Oxygen Saturation (SaO$_2$) < 95%
Active bleeding
Blood loss > 500 ml
Systolic blood pressure < 100 mm Hg or heart rate > 100 bpm
Adult respiratory distress syndrome (ARDS)

One way of measuring the effectiveness of the system's various critiquing messages is to examine the frequency with which the process of ordering blood products is terminated as a result of the feedback. During a 6-month period the ordering program was entered and then exited without an order 677 times. This was 12.9% of the total uses. We estimate that one-half of these exits represent decisions not to order blood products based on feedback from the program.

The program relies heavily on the integrated clinical database in the HELP system. It accesses data from: (1) the admitting department; (2) the clinical laboratory; (3) surgical scheduling; (4) the blood bank; and (5) the orders entered by nurses and physicians.

The blood-ordering program described above contains processes that support computerized critiquing. The program responds to interventions chosen by the physician by analyzing the order and, if appropriate, suggesting reasons to alter the therapeutic plan.

The process used by the blood-ordering program is different from that used in the alerting application in that it involves a dialogue with the user. As a result, the critique can provide a series of informational responses designed to assure that the user is fully aware of both the status of the patient and also the accepted guidelines governing blood product usage. Historically, physician use of generalized computerized order entry programs has been limited. However, modern order entry programs are being designed to encourage use by physicians. A part of this encouragement is based on the ability of these programs to critique orders. Physicians often appreciate the ability of an automated ordering system to give feedback on proper dosing and accepted care protocols as they make their intervention decisions. Opportunities for a constructive interaction between the computer and the clinician are clearly growing, and applications that critique medical decisions can contribute to this growth.

SUGGESTION SYSTEMS

The third category of computer applications designed to support medical decision-making is potentially the most interactive. This group of processes is designed to react to requests (either direct or implied) for assistance. These processes respond by making concrete suggestions concerning which actions should be taken next.

Unlike alerts, action oriented messages from these system are expected. Clinicians would typically call up a computer screen, enter requested data, and wait for suggestions from these systems before instituting a new therapy. Unlike critiquing systems, the physician need not commit to an order before the program applies its stored medical logic. Instead, the program conducts an interactive session with the user during which a suggestion concerning a specific therapeutic decision is sought. The system then reviews relevant data, including data that it has requested from the user, and formulates a suggestion for an intervention based on the medical knowledge stored in its knowledge base.

The example below is, in many ways, typical of suggestion systems. It functions in the realm of ventilator therapy and has been implemented in increasingly more sophisticated forms in intensive care settings at the LDS Hospital since 1987.

As a tertiary care setting, LDS Hospital sees a large number of patients with respiratory failure. One of the more difficult of these problems is that of Adult Respiratory Distress Syndrome (ARDS). This disease can complicate a number of other conditions including trauma, infectious disease, and shock. The usual therapy includes respiratory support while the underlying pulmonary injury heals. Unfortunately, overall mortality for ARDS had remained at about 50% for many years. For the subset of ARDS patients who manifest severe hypoxemia the mortality had been approximately 90%.

The study of computer protocols for ARDS patients was driven by research into the effectiveness of a new therapeutic intervention in this difficult disease. In the early 1980s research began to suggest that external membrane devices that bypassed the lungs to remove carbon dioxide (CO_2) directly from a patient's body might improve survival in the most severely ill of the ARDS patients. Physicians at the LDS Hospital wanted to study this new approach in a rigorously controlled clinical trial. They chose to do an experiment with a test group who received the external lung treatment and a control group who did not. However, the researchers were aware that the management of ARDS differed from patient to patient depending on the course the disease followed and the training and previous experience of the physicians and staff caring for the patient. For this reason, they decided to standardize care by strict adherence to predetermined treatment protocols.

At first, they developed a set of paper protocols. As the protocols became more complex, it became clear that they would be difficult to follow manually. Therefore it was decided to computerize them. The result was a set of computerized rules that were designed to direct, in detail, the management of patients in both the test and control branches of a study of extracorporeal CO_2 removal (ECCO$_2$R).[27-29] While the rules were designed initially for this research, they were soon made general enough that they could be used in the management of other patients requiring ventilatory support.

The protocols were created by a group of physicians, nurses, respiratory therapists, and specialists in medical informatics. The initial study period was to be 18 months. Subsequent development concentrated on first eliminating errors in protocol logic, second on extending its scope, and finally on reworking behavioral patterns in the intensive care setting so that the protocols could be effectively implemented.

The protocol system devised was used successfully during the ECCO$_2$R study. The study was terminated after 40 patients were treated, 21 with ECCO$_2$R and 19 with conventional therapy. At that time there were seven survivors in the ECCO$_2$R group (33%) and eight in the conventional therapy group (42%).[30] The study group concluded that there was no significant difference between ECCO$_2$R and conventional treatment of severe ARDS. However, the percentage of severely ill patients of this type who survived was usually less than 15% and the 42% survival in the control group was unexpected. The results led the researchers to suspect that the quality and uniformity of care provided through the use of computerized protocols had resulted in a significant improvement in patient outcomes.

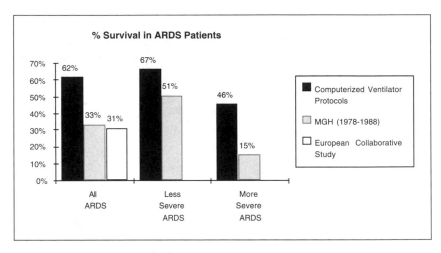

Fig. 4.1. Comparative results for groups managing ARDS patients.

As a consequence, development and study of these protocols has continued. Figure 4.1 summarizes the results of their use in the 111 LDS Hospital patients and compares these results to those of two other groups (Massachusetts General Hospital (MGH) and a group in Europe interested in the problem of treating ARDS).

It should be noted that here we have limited our example of systems for suggesting therapeutic interventions to a system that responds with a suggestion when the clinician has explicitly or implicitly requested one. Such a computerized decision support process is an area in which we are continuing to explore better ways to interact with clinicians and better ways to capture and encode protocol knowledge.

"DIAGNOSTIC" DECISION SUPPORT WITH THE HELP SYSTEM

The examples above have stressed different approaches to the activation of medical decision support logic and to the delivery of the resulting decisions to the computer user. Below we change our focus. One of the greatest challenges for a computerized medical decision system is to participate productively in the diagnostic process. Clinical diagnostic decision support systems (CDDSS) differ from the decision support systems described above. Decision support systems can draw attention to specific data elements and/or can synthesize therapeutic suggestions based on these elements. Such applications offer assistance in the basic recognition processes and can categorize patients by pathophysiologic condition. On the other hand, the diagnostic process is a preliminary step to making therapeutic interventions. Diagnostic decisions may require a system with different goals, interfaces, and decision algorithms than the applications previously described.

Two types of diagnostic applications are described below. They differ in the degree with which the developers have solved the problem of providing a clinically useful service. The first type represents modest applications that, using a set of raw clinical data, attempt to standardize various diagnostic categorizations that impact discrete therapeutic decisions. Three HELP system examples are discussed.

The second group of CDDSS comes from the family of applications that attempt to simulate the more extensive and flexible diagnostic behavior of physicians. Those discussed here are either preliminary research whose clinical application remains in the future or work in progress whose utility is a subject of ongoing evaluation. The status of these applications in terms of preliminary data and experience limited to a research and development environment is described.

PROVEN DIAGNOSTIC APPLICATIONS

A number of applications residing in the HELP system can, through the use of various diagnostic strategies, affect patient care. Below we describe three of these applications. The first is an application that evaluates patient data to detect adverse drug events. The second is a tool that recognizes nosocomial infections. The third is a computerized assistant that informs and advises physicians as they undertake the complex task of determining how to treat a patient with a possible infection.

Adverse Drug Events

Adverse drug events (ADEs) are defined by the World Health Organization as "any response to a drug which is noxious, unintended, and which occurs at doses normally used in man for the prophylaxis, diagnosis, or therapy of disease." ADEs can range in severity from drowsiness or nausea to anaphylaxis and death. It has been estimated that in the United States drug-related morbidity and mortality costs more than $136 billion per year.[31]

The process of recognizing ADEs differs from the drug monitoring at the time of drug dispensing that has become a standard part of computerized pharmacy systems. The alerting systems embedded in modern-day pharmacy dispensing systems typically evaluate ordered medications against a list of contraindications based on known allergies, expected reactions with other patient medications, or the information from the clinical laboratory that can be expected to affect the drugs given or the dosage of those medications. In contrast, the goal of an ADE detection system is to determine the existence of a drug reaction from the patient data collected during the routine documentation of patient care.

An ADE recognition subsystem has been implemented in the HELP system.[32-33] This ADE subsystem continuously monitors patients for the occurrence of an ADE. The system does so by inspecting the patient data entered at the bedside for signs of rash, changes in respiratory rate, heart rate, hearing, mental status, seizure, anaphylaxis, diarrhea and fever. In addition, data from the clinical lab, the pharmacy, and the medication charting applications are analyzed to determine possible ADEs.

The system evaluates all of the patients in the hospital and generates a daily computer report indicating which patients are possible ADE victims. A clinical pharmacist follows up on these patients and completes the evaluation using a verification program. This program provides a consistent method of completing the diagnostic process. A scoring system (the Naranjo method) is used to score the ADEs as definite (score 9), probable (score 5-8), possible (score 1-4), or unlikely (score 0).[34] The physicians caring for each patient are notified of confirmed ADEs by the pharmacist who does the evaluation.

The existence of an application for diagnosis of ADEs has increased the frequency with which these events are recognized and documented in the hospital setting. Using a voluntary reporting method, nine ADEs were recorded in the one-year period from May 1, 1988 to May 1, 1989. In the period from May 1, 1989 to May 1, 1990, while the program was in use, 401 adverse drug events were identified.

An additional effect of this program appears to be a reduction in the number of severe ADEs seen. During the year beginning in January of 1990, 41 ADEs occurred. In this time frame, physicians were notified of verified ADEs only if they were classified as severe or life threatening. In two subsequent periods (the year of 1991 and the year of 1992) early notification of physicians was practiced for all severities of ADE. Numbers of severe ADEs decreased to 12 and 15 during the follow-up time periods (p < 0.001).

In an effort to understand the impact of the drug reactions that were the target of this application, the costs of ADEs were examined. In studies that used the computer tools described above, investigators found that length of hospital stay for patients wtih ADEs was increased by 1.91 days and that costs resulting from the increased stay were $2,262. The increased risk of death among patients experiencing ADEs was 1.88 times.[35] Thus, the cost savings and impact on quality of care in reducing ADEs was substantial.

These tools leverage the fact that the majority of the data necessary for their function is available in HELP's integrated data base. They illustrate the potential for computerized diagnostic applications to impact patient care not just by assisting with the choice of interventions, but also by focusing clinical attention on those cases where the interventions chosen have put the patient at risk.

Nosocomial Infections

In the previous example a rule-based system was used to suggest the diagnosis of adverse drug events for a group of patients undergoing therapy in the hospital. Another application in use in the LDS Hospital is designed to recognize nosocomial, or hospital acquired infections.[36] The program serves a need recognized by the JCAHO, which requires ongoing surveillance for hospital-acquired infections.

The process of detecting nosocomial hospital infections serves a recognized clinical purpose. Control measures based on this information are believed to be important in interrupting the spread of hospital acquired infections. Evidence suggests that intensive surveillance programs may be linked to reduced rates of infection. However, the process can be expensive. Traditional techniques require infection control personnel to screen manually all appropriate patients on a routine basis.

The computerized surveillance system used in LDS Hospital relies on data from a variety of sources to diagnose nosocomial infections. Information from the microbiology laboratory, nurse charting, the chemistry lab, the admitting office, surgery, pharmacy, radiology and respiratory therapy are used. Once each day a report is produced detailing the computer's suggestions. This report can be used to followup the patients for whom there is evidence of nosocomial infection.

In studies done to compare the computer-based ascertainment of nosocomial infections to the traditional, manual approach, 217 patients were determined to be possible victims of hospital acquired infection (out of 4,679 patients discharged in a 2 month period). This included 182 patients identified by the computer and an overlapping 145 patients recognized by traditional means. Of these patients, 155 were confirmed to have nosocomial infections.

For the group of 155 patients, the computer's sensitivity was 90% with a false positive rate of 23%, while the infection control practitioners demonstrated a sensitivity of 76% and a false positive rate of 19%. When the hours required to use each approach were estimated, the computer-based approach was more than twice as efficient as the entirely manual technique.

The nosocomial infection tool, like the ADE recognition system, uses Boolean logic in a relatively simple diagnostic process. In an effort to extend the process of managing hospital acquired infections, an extension to the infection control system was developed. The goal of the enhancement was to predict which patients were likely to contract a nosocomial infection in the hospital in the future. The tool is based on different decision algorithms. Data from patients with infections acquired in the hospital were combined with data from a control set of patients, and a group of statistical programs were used to identify risk factors. Logistic regression using these risk factors was used in the development of tools that could estimate the risk of hospital-acquired infection for inpatients. The resulting system is capable of predicting these infections in 63% of the population who are ultimately affected.[37]

Recently, an assessment of a computerization of local clinician-derived practice guidelines used to recommend antibiotics has been conducted.[38] During a seven-year study, the fraction of patients who received antibiotics increased each year. However, the total cost of antibiotics decreased from almost 25% to only 13% of the total drug expenditures. Fewer doses of antibiotics and less expensive antibiotics were used as a result of the system's recommendations.

These computerized systems also monitor for that subset of surgical procedures for which prophylactic antibiotics are recommended (i.e., total hip replacement). For these procedures, antibiotics are often missed or given at the wrong time. In addition, once begun, these antibiotics are frequently not discontinued at the recommended time. In the absence of infection, a small number of doses is generally all that is required.

Based on computerized reminders, the number of patients who were given prophylactic antibiotics appropriately has increased from 40% of those who needed them to over 99%. In addition, the average number of antibiotic doses given as a part of prophylaxis decreased from 19 in the first year to only 5.3 doses at the end of the seven-year period. The accumulating experience suggests that computer-assisted support of antibiotic use can improve antibiotic use, reduce costs and stabilize the emergence of antibiotic-resistant pathogens.

Antibiotic Assistant

The third application is an example of a multipronged approach to the task of supporting medical decision making. As a part of ongoing research into the use of computers in medical care, the Infectious Disease Department at LDS Hospital has developed a tool to help clinicians make informed decisions concerning the administration of antibiotics.[39] The "antibiotic assistant" provides three basic services. First, it assembles relevant data for the physicians so they can determine whether a specific patient is infected and what sorts of interventions might be appropriate. Information such as the most recent temperature, renal function and allergies are presented. Second, the system suggests a course of therapy appropriate to that patient's condition. Finally, the program allows the clinician to review hospital experience with infections for the past 6 months and the past 5 years. One of the options of the program allows the clinician to review the logic behind the computer's suggestions while another presents brief monographs on the appropriate use of each antibiotic in the hospital formulary.

The diagnostic processes embedded in this application are derived from data extracted from the HELP system and analyzed on a monthly basis. The goal of the analysis is to define the probability of each potential pathogen as a causative agent for a certain class of patient. Six clinical variables are used in this process. These variables were identified through a statistical analysis of 23 proposed data elements. They include the site of infection, the patient's status (inpatient or outpatient), the mode of transmission (community or hospital acquired), the patient's hospital service, the patient's age and the patient's sex.

The result of this monthly analysis is an assessment of the likelihood of each pathogen for every combination of the patient-related variables. For example, once the first analysis is complete the percentage of hospital acquired bacteremias due to *Escherichia coli* in male patients age 50 or less who are on the cardiovascular service will be stored in the program's knowledge base. The analysis programs also evaluate susceptibility data to determine which antibiotics would probably cover the likely pathogens for each combination of patient variables.

This probabilistic knowledge is then filtered through a set of rules created by infectious disease experts. These rules adjust the output of the first phase to include criteria representing basic tenets of antibacterial therapy. For example, the susceptibility information garnered from the historical data would be updated to indicate that Amikacin should be used only for infections due to gram-negative organisms.

The resulting knowledge base is used by the antibiotic assistant program to make presumptive diagnoses of infectious organisms and to suggest treatments appropriate to these organisms. It remains up-to-date through monthly updates of its knowledge base. By offering the monographs and explanations mentioned above and by allowing the clinicians to browse its knowledge base, it provides large amounts of information in addition to its suggestions.

RESEARCH INTO COMPLEX DIAGNOSTIC APPLICATIONS

The systems described above have had a clear and measurable effect on improving health care provided in the hospital setting. The dream of even more sophisticated and inclusive systems were presented more than 30 years ago. In 1959, Ledley and Lusted described the application of methods from the realm of symbolic logic and statistical pattern recognition to problems in medicine.[40] They proposed that these tools be used to assist in the diagnostic process and in other problems involving medical decision-making. Computer systems were the enabling technology that was predicted to bring these tools to the bedside.

A variety of researchers have accepted the challenge of Ledley and Lusted and produced experimental systems designed to diagnose a variety of illnesses. A number of these systems are mentioned elsewhere in this book. Within the HELP system, researchers have created and tested several CDDSS. Two of these are described below.

An important portion of the value of computerized diagnostic tools lies in the development of well-designed models of the diagnostic process to assist in the complex clinical decision making tasks. Physicians clearly exercise their diagnostic knowledge not only when they assign a diagnostic label to a patient, but also during processes as diverse as reading medical reports and critiquing the clinical behavior of their peers. We give examples of experimental systems that: (1) assist with data collection; and (2) help assess the quality of medical reports.

The applications described below benefit from a long-standing interest in Bayesian techniques for probability revision among researchers using the HELP system. For more than 20 years the HELP system has contained a frame-based decision support subsystem capable of capturing and employing Bayes' equation to assess probabilistically the support for diagnoses provided by various combinations of clinical data.[8] Statistical approaches to decision support, such as those described in chapter 2 of this book, have been and continue to be key areas of research in the HELP medical informatics community.

Assisting Data Collection

Efforts to direct data collection in the HELP system have concentrated on the patient history. The goal has been to identify tools that could effectively collect a medical history appropriate for use in diagnostic decision support applications. While earlier efforts focused on history appropriate to a wide variety of diseases,[41] more recent efforts have focused on acquiring data bearing on pulmonary diseases.[42-43]

Three techniques for selecting questions were explored. The first was a simple branching questionnaire. This approach takes full advantage of the hierarchical relationship between more and less specific questions. For instance, if the question "Have you had chest pain with this illness?" was answered "Yes", then more specific questions such as "Is your chest pain brought on by exertion?" were asked. Alternately, if the answer to the first question was "No", the more specific questions would not be asked.

The second technique has been called Decision-driven Data Acquisition (DDA). With this technique, a frame-based, Bayesian, expert system analyzes all data available at any point in the patient interview. The individual disease frames determine which additional information is needed to evaluate the likelihood of the particular disease. Each frame proposes one or more questions. From this list, a supervisory program selects a group of five questions, which are then presented to the patient. The system passes through this cycle multiple times until criteria are met indicating that no additional data are needed.

A third approach has also been tested. It is similar to the DDA method except that it was adapted for use in a setting where the patient was not present at a computer terminal. The approach begins when a paper questionnaire containing screening questions is presented to a patient. The answers are entered into the computer and the patient's data are compared to the diagnostic frames. The questions are scored by a filtering process and then from 0 to 40 additional questions are printed for the patient to answer. After the patient answers these additional questions, the answers are entered into the computer and the process is completed.

The branching questionnaire mode of data collection and the DDA mode were tested on inpatients at the LDS Hospital. Fifty patients took a DDA managed history and 23 received a history managed by the branching questionnaire program. Figure 4.2 illustrates the results.

On average, the DDA mode took a significantly ($p < 0.05$) shorter time to run (8.2 minutes) and asked significantly fewer questions (48.8 questions) than did the branching questionnaire (19.2 minutes and 137 questions, respectively). The two-stage, paper questionnaire was tested separately on patients coming to the X-ray department for chest X-rays. It appeared to perform similarly to the interactive DDA mode. It should be noted that there was no significant difference between the techniques in terms of diagnostic accuracy. Using history alone, all three succeeded in placing the patient's correct disease in a five member differential diagnostic list from 70-88% of the time.

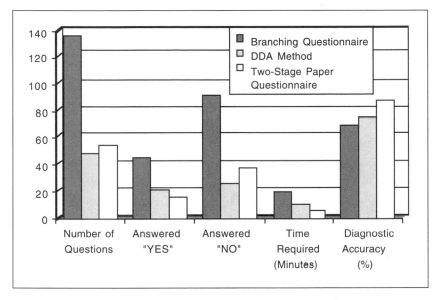

Fig. 4.2. A comparison of techniques for collecting the patient history.

Assessing the Quality of Medical Reports

A second example of an alternative use of diagnostic knowledge comes from a study of result reporting in the Radiology Department. The central goal of this project was to develop a technique for measuring the quality of X-ray reporting without requiring the review of radiographs by multiple radiologists. This is in contradistinction to typical approaches for evaluating the accuracy of radiologists. Typically, audit procedures in the Radiology department require multiple readings of a select set of X-rays.[44-48] The results of the repeated readings are used to define a "gold standard" for the films. Then the individual radiologists are compared to the gold standard.

The technique developed as a part of this project was based on a simple premise. Each examination was a test of the radiologist's accuracy. Instead of comparing the abnormalities reported to a standard formulated through multiple readings, the description in the report was evaluated in comparison to the patient's overall diagnostic outcome. In the case of chest X-rays the standard was the list of final diagnoses (ICD-9 codes) integrated into the patient's record at the time of discharge. The report generated by the radiologist was successful to the extent that it supported the process that led to one of the discharge diagnoses.

While a variety of algorithms can be used to link the findings represented in the X-ray report to the final diagnosis, we have demonstrated the success of a variation on Shannon Information Content in discriminating among physicians reading chest X-rays. Shannon Information Content[49] is a mathematical formalism for assessing the informational value of messages. We have modified it to provide a measure of the information produced by the radiologists as they interpret an X-ray. The assumption inherent in this usage is that the information contained in an X-ray report can be expected to alter the likelihood of the various diseases that a patient might have. Information Content is calculated from the change in probability of these diseases.

For this technique to work, a diagnostic system was required that was capable of discriminating among diseases producing abnormalities on the chest radiograph. The information content was calculated from the change in disease probability induced by the findings recorded in the chest X-ray report. A Bayesian system provided the required probabilities.

Our evidence for the success of this technique came from two studies. In the first we used expert systems technologies to demonstrate discrimination in a controlled experiment.[50] In this experiment five X-ray readers read an identical set of 100 films. The assessment produced by the diagnostic logic program gave results consistent with the differing expertise of the readers and similar to the results of a more standard audit procedure.

In a second study of this audit technique, we extended the test environment into the realm where we hope to use it clinically.[51] We tested a group of radiologists following their standard procedure for interpreting radiographs. Each chest X-ray was reviewed, the report dictated and transcribed only once as is typical with most radiologists' daily work. The goal of the study was to test the ability of a knowledge-based approach to measure the quality of X-ray reporting without requiring repeated reading of the radiographs.

This technique used a modified version of the Shannon Information Content measure and was designed to assess both the positive information contributed by X-ray findings relevant to a patient's disease and the negative information contributed by findings which do not apply to any of the patient's illnesses. X-ray readers were compared based on the bits of information produced. We used 651 chest X-ray reports generated by a group of radiologists that were compared to the patients' discharge diagnoses using a measure of information content. The radiologists were grouped according to whether they had received additional (post residency) training in chest radiology. The "Trained" radiologists produced 11% more information than the "Untrained" radiologists (0.664 bits as opposed to 0.589 bits, significant at $p < 0.005$).

The average information content calculated successfully discriminated these groups. However, it is an overall measure. Examination of the interaction between the groups of radiologists and disease subgroups indicates that the score can also discriminate at the level of different diseases ($p < 0.05$). This suggests that the technique might not only discriminate overall quality of X-ray interpretation, but it might also be of use at pinpointing the specific diseases for which an individual radiologist may be failing to generate effective information.

SUMMARY

In this chapter we have reviewed a number of hospital-based applications that provide medical decision support. These applications can be categorized in a variety of different ways. We have found it profitable to think of these systems in terms of their relationship to the data and of their interfaces with their users. These foci might be helpful to future system developers and implementers to reflect on the environment required for the success of decision support applications.

We have also attempted to emphasize the range of sophistication that can be found in a clinically operational CDDSS. Applications using simple logic can contribute a great deal to the quality of care provided in a clinical setting. Programs that use more complex techniques and that strive to provide the more sophisticated decisions associated with disease recognition can also contribute. Among the diagnostic applications currently functioning in hospital settings, those that focus on specific, limited diagnostic goals with a recognizable target audience have been more successful. General purpose diagnostic programs, while capable of producing interesting results, have yet to find an audience for which they can provide a routine, valued support function.

The lessons learned from the information systems used in hospitals are diffusing rapidly to the outpatient setting. Less expensive hardware, more flexible software, and an environment that increasingly values the efficiencies that computers can offer are encouraging the development of systems for a wide range of clinical settings. As this process occurs, the lessons gleaned by developers of CDDSS in the hospital setting should provide a springboard for the decision support systems of the future.

REFERENCES

 1. Bleich HL. The computer as a consultant. N Engl J Med 1971; 284:141-146.
 2. McDonald CJ. Protocol-based computer reminders, the quality of care and the non-perfectibility of medicine. N Engl J Med 1976; 295:1351-1355.
 3. Tierney WM, Overhage JM, McDonald CJ. Toward electronic records that improve care. Ann Intern Med 1995; 122:725-726.
 4. Clayton PD, Sideli RV, Sengupta S. Open architecture and integrated information at Columbia-Presbyterian Medical Center. MD Comput 1992; 9:297-303.
 5. Safran C, Herrmann F, Rind D et al. Computer-based support of clinical decision making. MD Comput 1990; 9:319-322.
 6. Teich JM, Geisler MA, Cimermann DE et al. Design considerations in the BWH ambulatory medical record: features for maximum acceptance by clinicians. Proc Annu Symp Comput Appl Med Care 1990:735-739.
 7. Geissbuhler A, Miller RA. A new approach to the implementation of direct care-provider order entry. Proc AMIA Fall Symp 1996:689-693.
 8. Kuperman GJ, Gardner RM, Pryor TA. HELP: A Dynamic Hospital Information System. New York: Springer-Verlag, 1991.
 9. Pryor TA, Clayton PD, Haug PJ et al. Design of a knowledge driven HIS. Proc Annu Symp Comput Appl Med Care 1987:60-63.
10. Gardner RM, Cannon GH, Morris AH et al. Computerized blood gas interpretation and reporting system. IEEE Computer 1975; 8:39-45.
11. Gardner RM. Computerized data management and decision making in critical care. Surg Clin N America 1985; 65:1041-1051.
12. Hulse RK, Clark SJ, Jackson JC et al. Computerized medication monitoring system. Am J Hosp Pharm 1976; 33:1061-1064.
13. Hripcsak G, Clayton PD, Pryor TA et al. The Arden syntax for medical logic modules. Proc Annu Symp Comput Appl Med Care 1990:200-204.
14. Haug PJ, Gardner RM, Tate KE et al. Decision support in medicine: examples from the HELP system. Comput Biomed Res 1994; 27:396-418.

15. Wheeler LA, Brecher G, Sheiner LB. Clinical laboratory use in the evaluation of anemia. JAMA 1977; 238:2709-2714.
16. Olsen DM, Kane RL, Proctor PH. A controlled trial of multiphasic screening. N Eng J Med 1976; 294:925-930.
17. Bradshaw KE, Gardner RM, Pryor TA. Development of a computerized laboratory alerting system. Comput Biomed Res 1989; 22: 575-587.
18. Tate KE, Gardner RM, Weaver LK. A computer laboratory alerting system. MD Comput 1990; 7:296-301.
19. Tate KE, Gardner RM. Computers, quality and the clinical laboratory: a look at critical value reporting. Proc Annu Symp Comput Appl Med Care 1993:193-197.
20. Tate KE, Gardner RM, Scherting K. Nurses, pagers, and patient-specific criteria: three keys to improved critical value reporting. Proc Annu Symp Comput Appl Med Care 1995:164-168.
21. Johnson DS, Ranzenberger J, Herbert RD et al. A computerized alert program for acutely ill patients. J Nurse Admin 1980; 10:26-35.
22. Kuperman GJ, Teich JM, Bates DW et al. Detecting alerts, notifying the physician, and offering action items: a comprehensive alerting system. Proc AMIA Fall Symp 1996:704-708.
23. Van Schoonhoven P, Berkmann EM, Lehman R, Fromberg R, eds. Medical Staff Monitoring Functions—Blood Usage Review. Chicago: Joint Commission on Accreditation of Hospitals, 1987.
24. Gardner RM, Golubjatnikov OK, Laub RM et al. Computer-critiqued blood ordering using the HELP system. Comput Biomed Res 1990; 23:514-528.
25. Lepage EF, Gardner RM, Laub RM et al. Improving blood transfusion practice: role of a computerized hospital information system. Transfusion 1992; 32:253-259.
26. Gardner RM, Christiansen PD, Tate KE et al. Computerized continuous quality improvement methods used to optimize blood transfusions. Proc Annu Symp Comput Appl Med Care 1993:166-170.
27. Sittig DF, Pace NL, Gardner RM et al. Implementation of a computerized patient advise system using the HELP clinical information system. Comput Biomed Res 1989; 22:474-487.
28. East TD, Henderson S, Morris AH et al. Implementation issues and challenges for computerized clinical protocols for management of mechanical ventilation in ARDS patients. Proc Annu Symp Comput Appl Med Care 1989:583-587.
29. Henderson S, East TD, Morris AH et al. Performance evaluation of computerized clinical protocols for management of arterial hypoxemia in ARDS patients. Proc Annu Symp Comput Appl Med Care 1989:588-592.
30. Morris AH, Wallace CJ, Menlove RL et al. A randomized clinical trial of pressure-controlled inverse ratio ventilation and extracorporeal

CO2 removal for adult respiratory distress syndrome. Am J Respir Crit Care Med 1994; 149:295-305.

31. Johnson JA, Bootman HL. Drug-related morbidity and mortality: a cost of illness model. Arch Intern Med 1995; 155:1949-1956.

32. Classen DC, Pestotnik SL, Evans RS et al. Computerized surveillance of adverse drug events in hospital patients. JAMA 1991; 266: 2847-2851.

33. Evans RS, Pestotnik SL, Classen DC et al. Development of a computerized adverse drug event monitor. Proc Annu Symp Comput Appl Med Care 1991:23-27.

34. Naranjo CA, Busto U, Sellers EM et al. A method for estimating the probability of adverse drug reacrions. Clin Pharmacol Ther 1981; 30:239-245.

35. Classen DC, Pestotnik SL, Evans RS et al. Adverse drug events in hospitalized patients: excess length of stay, extra costs, and attributable mortality. JAMA 1997; 277:301-306.

36. Evans RS, Larsen RA, Burke JP et al. Computer surveillance of hospital-acquired infections and antibiotic use. JAMA 1986; 256: 1007-1011.

37. Evans RS, Burke JP, Pestotnik SL et al. Prediction of hospital infections and selection of antibiotics using an automated hospital data base. Proc Annu Symp Comput Appl Med Care 1990:663-667.

38. Pestotnik SL, Classen DC, Evans RS et al. Implementing antibiotic practice guidelines through computer-assisted decision support: clinical and financial outcomes. Ann Int Med 1996; 124:884-890.

39. Evans RS, Classen DC, Pestotnik SL et al. A decision support tool for antibiotic therapy. Proc Annu Symp Comput Appl Med Care 1995:651-655.

40. Ledley RS, Lusted LB. Reasoning foundations of medical diagnosis. Science 1959; 130:9-21.

41. Warner HR, Rutherford BD, Houtchens B. A sequential Bayesian approach to history taking and diagnosis. Comput Biomed Res 1972; 5:256-262.

42. Haug PJ, Warner HR, Clayton PD et al. A decision-driven system to collect the patient history. Comput Biomed Res 1987; 20:193-207.

43. Haug PJ, Rowe KG, Rich T et al. A comparison of computer-administered histories. Proc Annu Conf—Am Assoc Med Syst Inf, Conf. 1988:21-25.

44. Herman PG, Gerson DE, Hessel SJ et al. Disagreements in chest roentgen interpretation. Chest 1975; 68:278-282.

45. Yerushalmy J. Reliability of chest radiology in the diagnosis of pulmonary lesions. Am J Surg 1955; 89:231-240.

46. Koran LM. The reliability of clinical methods, data, and judgments (second of two parts). N Engl J Med 1975; 293:695-701.

47. Rhea JT, Potsaid MS, DeLuca SA. Errors of interpretation as elicited by a quality audit of an emergency radiology facility. Radiol 1979; 132:277-280.

48. Raines CJ, McFarlane DV, Wall C. Audit procedures in the national breast screening study: mammography interpretation. J Can Assoc Radiol 1986; 37:256-260.
49. Shannon CE, Weaver W. The Mathematical Theory of Communication. Urbana: University of Illinois Press, 1949.
50. Haug PJ, Clayton PD, Tocino I et al. Chest radiography: a tool for the audit of report quality. Radiol 1991; 180:271-276.
51. Haug PJ, Pryor TA, Frederick PR. Integrating radiology and hospital information systems: the advantage of shared data. Proc Annu Symp Comput Appl Med Care 1992:187-191.

CHAPTER 5

Medical Education Applications

Michael J. Lincoln

This chapter reviews the use of clinical diagnostic decision support systems (CDDSS) for educating physicians, nurses, physician-assistants, and other medical professionals. The discussion of this topic is quite timely. Informatics technologies and decision support systems are now widely considered to be an important component of medical curricula and the medical education journal *Academic Medicine* now includes a regular informatics column.[1] Professional societies have also recognized this trend. The Society of General Internal Medicine and the American Board of Internal Medicine have recently established training standards for internists which include literature searching, use of decision making tools, and other informatics technologies. CDDSS can provide domain specific, case-based, clinical experiences for students to supplement actual patient experiences, which can be highly variable.

This chapter is divided into several parts: We begin by examining the reasons why medical CDDSS should be adopted in the curriculum, how the systems work, and how they may specifically act to enhance students' cognitive performance on medical cases. We then review the educational research on specific CDDSS. This chapter closes with a discussion of recommendations for further educational development and evaluation of CDDSS.

REASONS TO ADOPT CDDSS IN MEDICAL CURRICULA

Several factors favor the increased adoption of computerized CDDSS. First, students and graduate clinicians now face increasingly complex clinical information management tasks. CDDSS can aid them by storing complex medical information and retrieving it in a case-specific fashion. Second, the software and hardware platforms for such systems are being continuously improved and now work much better than they have in the past. In particular, computer equipment is becoming cheaper and easier to manage in campus and library networks. Third, faculty and students are becoming increasingly computer literate, and they are now enthusiastic about using information technologies for problem-based learning. We will briefly review these factors.

MANAGING THE LARGE VOLUME OF MEDICAL INFORMATION

The large volume of clinical information currently published is difficult for practitioners to manage.[2-4] For example, the National Library of Medicine's (NLM's) MEDLINE (MEDlars onLINE) database now contains 8.6 million records from 3,800 biomedical journals extending back to 1966, and 33,000 new articles are added per month (data from the NLM Web site, "www.nlm.nih.gov/databases/medline.html"). Society is demanding that this new medical information be applied efficiently and promptly in order to reduce medical care costs and improve results. One approach to this problem is called evidence-based medicine. Instead of basing clinical decisions primarily on opinion and "experience," evidence-based medicine is the systematic application of validated medical research to decision making in clinical practice.

While it appears straightforward, a variety of hurdles exist to the widespread adoption of evidence-based practices. First, busy physicians do not often have time or skills necessary to distill conflicting scientific evidence on a variety of topics. Experts, often recruited by professional societies and the government, must be recruited (and paid) to create usable practice guidelines out of primary data. Another hurdle is to disseminate the refined knowledge effectively. A final barrier is the actual adoption into individual clinical practices.

Knowledge engineers can incorporate practice guidelines into computable "knowledge bases" for CDDSS.[5] Nilasena and Lincoln did this, although they found it difficult to computerize written diabetes guidelines because they contained a variety of hidden contradictions and unrealistic requirements.[6] When guidelines are computerized they must be carefully examined and turned into actions and procedures which can be built into a computer program. Once the guidelines are incorporated into the computer, the system can greatly assist with the diffusion of the guidelines into practice. Without computer assistance this process can be slow, as Lomas and colleagues found when they studied Cesarean section guidelines in Canada.[7-8] Despite successful mass guideline dissemination, they found that Cesarean practices were virtually unchanged. Lomas and others have proposed strategies such as case-based tutoring, "academic detail men" (a la drug company salesmen), and the use of influential local opinion leaders to translate new physician knowledge into practices.

The people-based approaches proposed by Lomas and others can be expensive. CDDSS can also provide guideline-based, patient-specific prompts at relevant, actionable points in the care process.[6,9-10] For example the "Antibiotic Assistant" at the LDS Hospital in Salt Lake City is a decision support system which constantly monitors changing patterns of antibiotic susceptibility, bacterial pathogen profiles, and patient outcomes in infectious diseases.[11] Chapter 4 provides a description of this system and the cost savings that resulted from its use. The Antibiotic Assistant is an example of a decision support system which links to actual patient data and uses practice guidelines to actively assist physicians. CDDSS such as this can prompt physicians to apply the latest medical knowledge at actionable points in the patient care process while actually saving money.

SYSTEM AND HARDWARE IMPROVEMENTS

CDDSS have been improved substantially and have become more useful for education. One key improvement has been the growth in complexity and domain coverage of the systems' knowledge bases. The first such systems were often focused in specific, narrow domains, such as abdominal pain diagnosis.[12] Such systems were quite important, but not necessarily suitable for general curricular use. CDDSS which cover entire specialities, such as internal medicine, are now readily available. The inference engines used by the CDDSS have also been improved, especially as the available processing power of the hardware has increased. As Gordon Moore, the cofounder of Intel Corporation, noted, hardware processing power doubles approximately every 18 months ("Moore's Law"). These improvements have allowed the use of increasingly complex mathematical models for processing knowledge bases. System developers have also taken advantage of this processing power to build in powerful teaching tools, not just for browsing, but also to analyze and compare potential work-up strategies. Taken together, these improvements have allowed today's CDDSS to work faster and better.

PROBLEM-BASED LEARNING AND INCREASED COMPUTER LITERACY

As medical schools adopt problem-based learning curricula, many are considering how to incorporate medical informatics technologies.[5] Cognitive research indicates that students will improve their performance when they are able to practice on cases in particular domains and receive performance feedback.[13-16] These findings are one reason why problem-based learning curricula attempt to provide students with standardized problem experiences in appropriate training domains. Problem-based learning can be quite costly because the faculty resources for small group teaching sessions and standardized patients (individuals trained to portray specific patient cases) are quite expensive. Many programs therefore emphasize student self-learning and group teaching. CDDSS can offer student-centered, problem-based learning in a cost-effective manner. The systems can provide case analysis and generate simulated cases in targeted training domains.

THE NATURE OF MEDICAL CDDSS

Teachers must know how CDDSS work. The information will partly determine how they employ the system's teaching functions, and will also influence the range of evaluation options. CDDSS can make diagnostic, therapeutic, and prognostic assessments. As described in chapter 2, these systems typically include two basic architectural components: a knowledge base and an inference engine. The knowledge base is the collection of expert medical knowledge used by the system, consisting of literature, statistics, disease-finding relationships, and other forms of compiled knowledge. The inference engine is the set of computer algorithms used to process patient findings in relation to the knowledge base.

KNOWLEDGE BASES

Understanding a bit about CDDSS knowledge bases is a key to understanding their content and using them for teaching. The author has worked as a knowledge engineer for the Iliad and QMR systems.

In the knowledge engineering process, the development team first defines the content of a new knowledge base[17] and selects expert consultants. Frequent knowledge engineering meetings are scheduled for each expert. Iliad covers about 15 broad domains, and we have found that two full-time knowledge engineering conference rooms are required. Knowledge base components are often called profiles (QMR) or frames (Iliad). Work on a specific frame (e.g., Perinephric Abscess) begins with a literature review to determine the relevant disease findings and their frequencies (e.g., sensitivity and specificity). Other knowledge sources typically include the clinical information system[18] or national databases (e.g., the National Center for Health Statistics data). The experts' domain knowledge is used extensively. Using these resources the team identifies the diagnostic features of the disease. For instance diagnostic features of perinephric abscess would include fever, chills, flank tenderness, elevated white blood cell count. The features for each disease are entered in a database record called a frame or a profile. Diagnostic features are coded and entered in a separate system vocabulary file called a data dictionary.

The core of each profile or frame is a list of diagnostic findings for a given disease. Iliad is a probabilistic Bayesian system and therefore each finding's specificity and sensitivity must be defined. Iliad knowledge engineers group the conditionally dependent findings into subsidiary frames called clusters.[19] These clusters are imbedded in the main profile and referenced by their sensitivity and specificity for the profile. QMR uses a heuristic algorithm that requires that each finding include information on what is called its "evoking strength" and "frequency." Evoking strength measures how strongly the presence of the finding should trigger or evoke consideration of the disease, a bit like positive predictive value. The expert uses the medical literature to assign a value of 0 to 5 for the evoking strength of each finding, with 0 used for nonspecific findings and 5 used for pathognomonic findings. Finding frequency is analogous to sensitivity, and is described using a 1-5 scale.[20-21] The resulting Iliad frame looks like a set of nested disease descriptions referenced (mostly) by probabilities. The QMR disease profile is a flat list of findings referenced by evoking strength and frequency. Additional information is added to this basic structure. For example, Iliad includes treatment profiles and QMR contains linkages describing how one disease may cause or predispose to another.

Knowledge base validation is a critical step and involves both analyzing actual cases and performing mathematical analyses of frame reliability.[19,20,22] Experts must adjust the finding probabilities, scores, or relationships to correct faulty performance. Knowledge engineering is expensive. About 150,000 person-hours have been expended on the development of Iliad's knowledge base; and at least 50 person-years (over 100,000 person hours) on QMR's knowledge base(Personal communication, Barry Blumenfeld MD, First DataBank). This accounts for about 115 to 165 person-hours per disease profile or frame. Managing this large effort requires knowledge engineering tools such as QMR's KAT (Knowledge Acquisition Tool)[20,21] and Iliad's KESS (Knowledge Engineering Support System).[17]

INFERENCE ENGINES

Inference engines used in medical CDDSS include Bayesian, rule-based, heuristic, neural networks, and Bayesian belief networks (see chapters 2 and 7 for more details on these types of inference engines). The type of inference engine and the corresponding knowledge base design can influence teaching use. For example, Bayesian systems predict the posterior probability of diagnoses based on the prior disease probabilities and the sensitivity and specificity of confirmed patient findings.[23] Such systems assess the information content of potential confirmatory findings during a work-up and use this information to assess the student's work-up.[24] Rule-based systems process sets of Boolean "if-then" rules. Forward and backward chaining of rules may be used to conclude a diagnosis and provide diagnostic explanations for teaching.[25] Heuristic systems such as QMR include quasi-statistical measures. QMR's disease profiles list the potential disease findings and the evoking strength of each finding for the given disease and the expected frequency of each finding in the disease. These measures can be used to evaluate alternative work-up strategies and to teach students the key points in a case which evoke the differential diagnosis. A key teaching function in each of these systems is provided by simply browsing the knowledge base (e.g., decision rules or disease profiles). Neural networks are perhaps less amenable to browsing or providing diagnostic explanations than some of the other systems, although Bayesian belief networks (which are often created as reformulations of traditional Bayesian representations) provide many of the same browsing and explanation capabilities of traditional systems.[26]

HOW CDDSS CAN ENHANCE CLINICAL PROBLEM SOLVING

Commercially available CDDSS typically offer consultation, simulation, and browsing modes. The consultation mode is used to diagnose or treat an actual patient. The simulation mode provides a vicarious patient encounter. The browsing mode uses the knowledge base as an electronic textbook of medicine. Teachers should use these modes in reference to knowledge about how students develop medical expertise.

How Students Develop Medical Expertise

Elstein and colleagues significantly advanced research in medical problem solving. They found that early hypothesis generation and hypothesis-centered deductive reasoning were key elements of the diagnostic process for both diagnostic experts and novices.[13-14] The findings of Elstein et al. suggested that medical experts performed better than novices because they possessed more domain-specific knowledge. Expert physicians used this knowledge to be highly selective in acquiring subsequent data. In fact, although they achieved superior results, the experts were typically less "thorough" than novices. Elstein et al. interpreted these results to mean that thoroughness of data collection was not correlated with accuracy of data interpretation. These important findings were in sharp contrast to the views of earlier researchers, who held that general abilities or learned strategies were the hallmarks of expertise.[27] These older views are remarkably persistent; today's professors often admonish students to "do a complete work-up" before making a diagnosis. Elstein et al. found little evidence that students heed such strategies, or that they are effective. They instead documented the overwhelming importance of domain-specific knowledge and data interpretation. Since then, other researchers have confirmed and extended these basic findings.[28-31]

Kassirer and Kopelman have taken a clinically-based approach to understanding medical problem solving. They analyzed a series of 40 cases which were later published in *Hospital Practice*.[32] Each case transcript consisted of a case narrative and an accompanying narrative of an expert discussant "thinking aloud" about the case. The analysis assessed the nature of the case, the number and type of any diagnostic errors, and the outcomes of the errors. The resulting taxonomy of errors included: (1) faulty triggering of hypotheses (failure to evoke or generate the hypothesis); (2) development of an incorrect context or problem space to represent the problem (e.g. framing the case as a collagen vascular disease instead of a neoplasm); (3) faulty gathering, interpretation, or processing of information; (4) inadequate verification of the diagnosis (failing to prove the main diagnosis with adequate certainty and/or failing to rule out the competitors); and (5) a catch-all category called "no fault." Their approach possessed a face validity for clinicians and also corroborated the results of the research on diagnostic problem solving. Kassirer and Kopelman illustrated the sometimes serious consequences of diagnostic errors (e.g., delayed chemotherapy for cancer, unnecessary nephrectomy). Voytovich and colleagues also commented on the importance of the first error category, faulty hypothesis triggering.[33] Voytovich and colleagues found that an aspect of consultants' efficacy may be their ability to "take a fresh look" at the patient and trigger appropriate hypotheses which have been overlooked.

Implications for Student Education via CDDSS

These research results indicate that we faculty do not necessarily serve students well by teaching them to always "do complete work-ups" or to analyze the various "congenital, acquired, infectious, atheromatous...." causes of a condition. We should instead provide domain-specific case experiences with performance feedback. This experience is expensive to provide. Students slow down attending physicians who are now under more pressure to work efficiently, hospital and clinic space is costly to build, and standardized patients (actors) are expensive to implement. In consultation mode, a CDDSS can be used to identify important diagnostic findings and to propose subsequent work-up steps. The systems can provide prompt feedback that faculty may sometimes be too busy to provide. CDDSS can also assist students in evoking appropriate diagnostic hypotheses, thus correcting another key source of diagnostic errors.[33] The systems can interactively assist and correct students as they perform the key diagnostic steps of formulating appropriate hypothetico-deductive inquiries and interpreting patient data.

The research results also imply that students should receive training on a representative range of patient cases that span their intended training domains. Student experiences with real cases are often uncontrolled, and the tertiary care case mix at most training centers may be atypical compared to the cases students' will see when they enter clinical practice settings after completion of training.[34] For example, we examined our students' internal medicine clerkship logs at the University of Utah. Our students typically experienced less than 15% of the diseases found on their junior clerkship goals and objectives, and only five percent saw a case of community-acquired pneumonia. If student experiences are not representative, they may later fail to evoke appropriate diagnostic hypotheses, mis-estimate probabilities, pursue expensive, but unlikely, diagnostic propositions, and select expensive diagnostic tests instead of more cost-effective examinations. CDDSS can provide realistic case simulations to fill in gaps in student case experiences and thereby correct these errors.

EXAMPLES OF CDDSS IN MEDICAL EDUCATION

CDDSS have been incorporated into medical education programs in several ways: (1) in a case simulation mode to provide additional case-based diagnostic experiences for students; (2) as electronic textbooks which provide compiled disease information; and (3) in their consultation modes to assist students in their routine clerkship activities and as part of specific problem-based exercises. CDDSS and other informatics applications have also been part of elective or required educational experiences in medical informatics. The next few pages describe some specific examples of broad-based and more narrowly focused CDDSS. When there has been research on the effects of these systems on student learning, the results of these studies are discussed. The first three systems described, QMR, Iliad and DXplain, are comprehensive systems covering the domain of internal medicine, and the others are targeted to specific diseases.

QUICK MEDICAL REFERENCE (QMR)

The CDDSS known as Quick Medical Reference (QMR) covers the domain of internal medicine and was developed as an outgrowth of the CADUCEUS/Internist-I project by Miller, Masarie, and Myers at the University of Pittsburgh School of Medicine.[35,36] The system was acquired by Camdat, a company now owned by First DataBank Inc., a division of the Hearst Corporation (http://www.firstdatabank.com). (Dr. Miller continues his research on what we have referred to in chapter 1 as R-QMR, the research version of QMR). QMR runs on IBM-PC compatible microcomputers under Microsoft Windows and requires an Intel 80486 or better machine with at least 4 megabytes of free disk space and eight megabytes of random access memory. A Macintosh version is also available. The system covers 680 disorders in internal medicine and the data dictionary contains 5,000 medical findings.

QMR was originally designed to operate in three modes: as an electronic textbook, as a "spreadsheet" for testing simple diagnostic concepts, and in the form of an expert consultant. A case simulation mode was added later.[37] Consultation mode users may enter patient findings in an open-ended manner or in an alternative confirmatory mode that focuses on a diagnosis. In these modes, users can examine QMR's suggested best work-up strategy, browse disease profiles (lists of diagnostic findings associated with a disease), review diagnostic codes, and browse the knowledge base. Users may also invoke a "filter" function which creates "rule-in" or "rule-out" criteria for any selected disease.

QMR's simulated cases are created by a sort of case analysis process running in reverse. This process generates the simulated case using the knowledge base's finding frequency information for the selected disease. In simulation mode, users can always use the textbook mode to examine lists of disease findings, to view finding frequencies and evoking strengths, and to obtain literature references which were selected by the knowledge engineers.

Several researchers have evaluated QMR's role in education. Miller and Schaffner reported in 1982 that the CADUCEUS/Internist-I and QMR systems had been used in student education for ten years at the University of Pittsburgh in a course titled "The Logic of Problem-Solving in Clinical Diagnosis".[38] The course was jointly taught by two "clinicians" and two "logicians" who alternated their didactic lectures and problem-solving exercises. They covered formal diagnostic reasoning models, the medical problem-solving theories of cognitive psychologists, and the work of decision analysts. Students also learned about the logical structures and algorithms used by expert systems. CADUCEUS was used in a consultation mode during the problem-solving exercises. In these sessions the instructors compared and contrasted the approach taken by clinician-discussants and the computer program. In an evaluation of this course, students rated it highly (a mean rating of 6.5 on an 8 point scale).

Seven years later Miller and Masarie updated readers on the use of QMR for medical education.[39] They discussed their use of QMR to meet curricular objectives for informatics education. For example, they had created a senior student rotation in medical informatics and knowledge engineering. Students on the rotation participated in the literature search, recruited a faculty expert, and organized and participated in the actual knowledge engineering sessions. They also described the development of QMR's patient simulator mode, which was specifically designed for teaching. Another faculty objective which Miller described was to provide students with a QMR textbook mode to access relevant medical information. This modality included various ways to display and stratify disease profiles, review other diseases that are associated with a given disease, and review literature references retrieved through a link to MEDLINE via the NLM's Grateful Med program. Finally, the authors described how the diagnostic spreadsheet and expert consultant modes were created from the original CADUCEUS/Internist-I model. First DataBank is continuing to develop different modes of QMR delivery, including an Internet version of QMR.

ILIAD

Iliad is a CDDSS originally developed at the University of Utah by Dr. Homer R. Warner and colleagues (including this author), and codeveloped by Applied Medical Informatics (http://www.ami-med.com/), a company which is now part of Mosby Year Book Inc.'s Consumer Health Division. Iliad version 4.5 was released in March, 1997, and runs on Macintosh and Windows microcomputers with at least 16 MB of random access memory and 15 MB of free disk space. The Iliad 4.5 knowledge base covers 930 diseases in the fields of internal medicine, pediatrics, dermatology, psychiatry, obstetrics and gynecology, peripheral vascular diseases and sleep disorders. The system's data dictionary contains 1500 syndromes and treatment protocols and 11,900 findings which describe the diagnostic elements used in the system. Digital images are now linked with the knowledge base. Iliad's functions include diagnostic consultation, case simulation, and a browsing mode. Treatment information is available for each disease covered by the system. Iliad was originally derived from part of the HELP system's knowledge base and inference engine (see chapter 4 regarding HELP). The knowledge base has been evaluated by mathematical analyses using a variety of test cases, as well as by comparison with gold standard expert diagnoses.[19,24,40]

Medical Student Teaching

In our teaching, we have chosen to use Iliad's simulation mode as a primary intervention. We have not systematically evaluated Iliad's consultation or browsing modes except for assessing student-perceived efficacy. In these studies, Iliad's nonsimulation functions were perceived favorably compared to other standard methods of teaching, such as books, journals, lectures and medical rounds.[41-42] Iliad simulated cases may be created in one of two ways. First, the user may choose to simulate de novo a selected (or randomly chosen) disease from the knowledge base. This type of simulation is similar to QMR's because it is created from the probabilistic information in the knowledge base. The alternative method is for faculty to enter actual cases from patient charts in consultation mode and then turn them into simulations.[24] A Student Interface Case Files (SICF) Manager program allows faculty to create time-dependent sequences of simulations, keyed to individual student identifiers, that can be used for training or testing students.[24]

Students who open a simulated learning case first see the simulated chief complaint and any associated complaints which the faculty have selected. The system selects one of two initial modes for the work-up. If any diagnostic probability on Iliad's differential is greater than a probability threshold of 0.05 (this may be adjusted), the student must select at least one diagnostic hypothesis before proceeding with the work-up. Otherwise the student may acquire additional diagnostic information without reference to any particular diagnostic hypothesis. This "free questions" mode is not scored or evaluated by Iliad. When the threshold is later exceeded, the student must enter one or more diagnostic hypotheses and reference each subsequent diagnostic inquiry to a hypothesis. This process teaches students that they must form early diagnostic hypotheses and then use these hypotheses to direct their work-ups. Students frame history, physical exam, and lab queries. Iliad responds with positive or negative answers (or numerical values, in the case of certain labs). Students may view Iliad's differential diagnosis at any time or choose to display it continuously as the work-up proceeds. Students may also browse the contents of the knowledge base to review diagnostic features and diseases. Iliad can stratify the work-up by displaying the findings that are explained or unexplained by diseases on the differential. The system also shows the information content that alternative findings can provide. Finally, Iliad's "Cheat Menu" allows the student to obtain "free questions" one at a time, or even view the name of the correct diagnosis.

During a simulated case work-up Iliad provides several numerical scores that can be used to evaluate student performance. The Hypothesis Score assesses the matching of the student's best hypothesis to Iliad's best hypothesis at each stage in the work-up. This score is a function of the posterior probability Iliad assigns to the student's selected best diagnosis, divided by the posterior probability Iliad assigns its own best hypothesis. This score ranges from 1.0 (the student has selected Iliad's best hypothesis) to 0 (the student has selected a totally unsupported hypothesis). The Findings Score measures the information content of each work-up step. Iliad's information content for any finding obtained during a work-up is calculated as the likelihood ratio (sensitivity divided by false positive rate) divided by a function of cost (alternative formulations have been evaluated, see Guo et al.[40]). The Findings Score is the ratio of the information content of the student's chosen finding divided by that of the best finding that Iliad would select. This score ranges from 1 (the student has selected the best findings Iliad could propose) to 0 (the student has selected findings which are totally irrelevant for the disease being pursued). Iliad can provide mean Hypothesis and Findings Scores for the work-up and also display the total costs of student-selected diagnostic procedures and tests. These scores approximate the type of feedback that a faculty member might provide. However, the Iliad model is simplified as compared to faculty feedback because the system does not consider diagnostic urgency or the risks of procedures and tests.

A final teaching feature that is incorporated for use during simulated cases run in learning mode is the "graduation march", which reinforces an adequate diagnostic performance. When the student has (1) selected the correct diagnosis as the top hypothesis and (2) documented enough evidence so that Iliad's probability for that diagnosis reaches the "treatment threshold" (normally set at a posterior probability of 0.95), the Mormon Tabernacle Organ is heard playing the "graduation march" (Dr. Robert Cundick's father was formerly the chief organist for the Tabernacle Choir). As the march plays, a congratulatory screen appears.

Iliad also provides a simulation-testing mode which we have employed together with the learning mode in order to evaluate Iliad's educational effects. The evaluations required carefully controlled experimental designs for using the learning and testing cases. The SICF Manager was used to create these designs as it allowed us to create a unique sequence of Iliad training simulations for each student. The main difference in using simulations in the testing mode compared to the learning mode is that in the testing mode all the teaching tools and scoring feedback are withheld. The student receives the patient's chief complaint and pursues the work-up in a normal fashion except for the lack of feedback. When students attain a so-called treatment threshold (a posterior probability of 0.95), they are instructed to close the cases. After the cases are sealed, the system generates summary scores and provides immediate feedback. Students can save unfinished cases and resume them later.

Analysis of the results of learning and testing mode simulations was automated by a program called CaseStats. The tool can process single cases or batches of cases (e.g., all of the cases in the "Iliad-trained" condition in one batch). CaseStats creates summary tables of several performance measures including the number of correct diagnoses, average Hypothesis and Findings Scores, the total Cost of the work-up, and the number of findings obtained. CaseStats provides certain statistical analyses automatically and provides tables which can be loaded into a database management system or used with another statistical package.

Evaluation of Use of Iliad with Medical Students

This author and other investigators have evaluated Iliad's training efficacy.[24,41-45] One detailed study involved 100 junior medical students assigned to their internal medicine clerkships at three Salt Lake City teaching hospitals.[24] All students received training in Iliad's simulation mode and subsequent user support. Students received Simulation Training Set cases from either a relatively high prevalence set of diseases (Common level of this variable) or relatively low prevalence (Uncommon) set of training cases. For example, congestive heart failure was one of the Common cases and analgesic nephropathy was a relatively low prevalence disease, and was included in the Uncommon set. These diseases were selected because they were identified as high priorities for student training on the Clerkship Director's goals and objectives. All students were subsequently tested on both Common and Uncommon cases. This created the Simulation Test Set independent variable. Students completed four training cases and four test cases (one per week) during four weeks of their six week rotation. Each case required about 30-45 minutes, and students were instructed to complete them without assistance. The SICF Manager was used to create a counterbalanced design for the student assignments.

The results showed that students who were Trained in Uncommon disease cases committed significantly fewer Final Diagnostic Errors (mean = 10.9%) than students who were trained in Common diseases (mean = 21.7%). A planned comparison of the students' results on the Final Diagnostic Errors variable also indicated that students made more errors on the Uncommon cases where they were not trained (mean = 21.7%) than the average of the other three conditions (mean = 7.7%). The results for the Posterior Probability dependent variable were also significant. A planned comparison of the mean student performance on this variable for the Uncommon cases in which they were trained (73.6%) was significantly higher than the other three conditions. The results on the Hypothesis Score variable were not significant. Pearson correlations showed that the correlations between the dependent variables were significantly correlated within replications (there were two six week rotations) but less correlated between replications.

The results showed improved student performance on tests of the relatively Uncommon cases if they had previous training in them, but not the Common cases. Students may have already been well versed on the Common case subject matter or Iliad training might have been ineffective for those cases. The Common cases may have simply been too easy (a ceiling effect). Iliad training and testing consumed only a small fraction of teaching during the six week rotations, and a more intensive program might have shown stronger effects. The study was also limited because there was no Iliad-untrained group, and because the students' real case experiences were not controlled.

Nurse Practitioner Training

The University of Utah Nursing Informatics faculty evaluated Iliad in their Nurse Practitioner Program. Nurse practitioners must develop enhanced diagnostic medical skills and Iliad was viewed as a cost-effective way to provide case experience. The nursing faculty trained 16 nurse practitioner students using a design similar to the one used for the medical students. They used a different set of simulated cases that better matched what these students would later see on their clinical rotations. The cases were derived from two content domains: Abdominal Pain cases (e.g., viral gastroenteritis) and Chest Pain cases (e.g., community-acquired pneumonia). The dependent variables were Diagnostic Errors, Cost, Posterior Probability, and Average Hypothesis Score. This study controlled for the students' real case experiences by means of a Case Specific Experience Inventory (CSEI).[46] The CSEI independent variable was used as a covariate to explain and statistically control within-condition variability in performance.

The results showed a significant effect for the Test Domain main effect. An examination of the means showed that the students had more previous experience with chest pain cases (CSEI score mean = 11.67) than abdominal pain cases (mean = 6.76). These results indicated that students might perform better on the simulated chest pain cases. The Final Diagnostic Errors dependent variable was not statistically significant, although the means were in the hypothesized direction (Diagnostic Errors were 6% in the Trained condition and 23% in the Untrained condition). A biserial correlation between the CSEI and Diagnostic Error variables showed that prior case experience was marginally significant for the chest pain cases [r = .4, p < 0.10] but not statistically significant for the abdominal pain cases [r = -.15, p > 0.10]. The Posterior Probability dependent variable was also not significantly different between the chest pain cases (mean = 0.74) and the abdominal pain cases (mean = 0.80). Prior case experience did not predict which students would perform better. Interestingly, the analysis of the Cost independent variable was significant and showed that students who trained and tested on abdominal pain cases spent substantially more on their work-ups (mean = $230) than students in the other three conditions (mean = $75 to $132 depending on the condition).

The nurse practitioner study demonstrated that prior case experience had some predictive value for student performance on Diagnostic Errors, but not on Posterior Probability. While some of the main effects were in the hypothesized directions, they were not significant. This may have occurred because of the small number of subjects (a type II error) or large error variance. The latter might have occurred because the nurse practitioner students had more highly variable prior experiences than the more uniformly trained medical students (some were experienced ICU nurses and others were recent undergraduates).

Physician Assistant Training

The Utah Physician Assistant Program and several other PA programs have used Iliad in their curricula. PA students also have variable prior experience (e.g., former Armed Services medic, nurses, ski patrolman, emergency medical technician). The Utah PA Program has implemented Iliad training as part of a comprehensive medical informatics curriculum for their students. Students complete simulated cases and use Iliad's consultation mode on real cases that they encounter in small group discussions and clinics. The students have not been formally evaluated to assess Iliad's training effects. Students have completed questionnaires to assess their satisfaction with the Informatics curriculum and Iliad.

DXPLAIN

DXplain is a CDDSS that covers general internal medicine. The system was developed by Dr. G. Octo Barnett and colleagues at Harvard Medical School's Laboratory of Computer Science[47,48] (http://lcsguide.mgh.harvard.edu/lcshome/dxplain.htm). DXplain's knowledge base contains 5,000 diagnostic findings and covers approximately 2,000 disease entities. The system's inference engine uses a modified form of Bayes' theorem to process diagnostic findings. DXplain users may enter findings and diagnose cases, focus on a particular complaint and explain the diseases that may cause it, review literature on the diseases in the knowledge base, and perform other useful functions. An interesting and unique feature of the system is that stand-alone programs (e.g., an electronic medical record system) can access DXplain through Web sockets to process diagnostic queries. DXplain was originally created in a version that ran at Massachusetts General Hospital and a nationally available version was available over the AMA/NET, an online network no longer in existence. DXplain is available in a stand-alone form for use under Microsoft DOS or Windows and is the only CDDSS now available in a Web-based format. Schools or individuals may license DXplain through the Laboratory of Computer Science.

DXplain consultations require the user to enter principal findings such as the patient's age, sex, and chief complaint. Using the Web version, these entries are submitted via forms. The Web response time is a bit slower than a stand-alone system such as Iliad or QMR, but it is quite acceptable. After entering initial complaints the user adds any other relevant complaints. Like the other systems we have discussed, DXplain maps their queries to a standard vocabulary and the user chooses the closest match. After entering the major complaints the user may request DXplain to generate potential diagnoses. The users can also ask DXplain to show the findings which tend to confirm a particular diagnosis or the findings which could be obtained to work-up a diagnosis. The system also provides a means for browsing the knowledge base in a textbook mode.

The author has used DXplain as part of a Medical Informatics course taught in Finland at the University of Helsinki Department of General Practice and has proposed using the system in the University of Utah's new problem-based curriculum (which is now being created). Dr. Barnett and colleagues at Harvard have employed DXplain as one component of a comprehensive, problem-based curriculum reform.[49-50]

PATHMASTER

PATHMASTER was developed at the Yale University School of Medicine in order to teach histopathologic differential diagnosis.[51] The system's current domain is liver diseases, although it is designed to be extensible to other domains. PATHMASTER was designed to teach students a "criteria-based" approach and "disease-directed analysis." In the criteria-based approach students are taught a systematic method to gather diagnostic features by anatomical systems and subsystems and to examine the relevant attributes of each anatomic sub-component of a pathological specimen. Students who examine a liver slide might discover bile duct fibrosis to be an important sign of portal triad disease. The system would then prompt a search for related portal triad findings such as bile pigment and cellular infiltrates. After the portal triad examination was complete, the system would prompt students to examine other sub-components of the liver slide such as the condition of the cellular parenchyma and blood vessels. The developers call this procedure "systematic analysis". In "disease-directed analysis," students selectively acquire features to confirm or to rule-out each plausible diagnosis evoked by the initial analysis.

The PATHMASTER system uses the generalized and disease-directed strategies described above in its own internal processing. The system employs Bayesian analysis to determine the posterior probability of contending diseases. Each PATHMASTER disease profile contains the disease's a priori probability, a list of findings occurring in the disease, and the sensitivities and specificities for each finding. The system supplements the systematic analysis and disease-directed analysis approaches by means of a simple analysis of the information content of as yet unobtained findings, along with additional weighting for the system or sub-system being analyzed. For example, a finding of female vs. male sex might (by itself) have a higher information content for the diagnosis of primary biliary cirrhosis than a certain portal triad feature. However, if other portal triad abnormalities have been found, an additional weight is given towards "systematically" obtaining the other features. This feature is said to reduce the tendency of the system to "jump around" excessively among different diseases during a case analysis.

The PATHMASTER system is designed to promote students' knowledge of specific disease-finding links by means of its "systematic analysis" mode. PATHMASTER switches (at a mathematically determined point) from systematic analysis to a disease-directed strategy, much as a real expert does. Students may learn the a priori disease frequencies of liver disease, perhaps correcting unrealistic expectations concerning base rates. Users can also select a key pathologic or clinical feature (e.g., presence of anti-mitochondrial antibodies) and view a probabilistic differential diagnosis of that key feature. This capability can teach domain-specific links between key pathophysiologic features and the diseases in the knowledge base. The developers of PATHMASTER have discussed the need to evaluate this and similar systems in teaching settings.

UNIVERSITY OF RENNES COMPUTER-ASSISTED INSTRUCTION PROGRAM

Fontaine and colleagues at Rennes have developed a "Computer-Assisted Instruction (CAI)" program.[52] The system uses the SUPER knowledge engineering environment and runs on "several knowledge bases;" although the exact domains are not specified. This CDDSS was designed to teach students by means of case simulations. CAI contains an author module for cases and can create cases using the information in the knowledge base. A pedagogical and a student module are subsequently required to run the case simulations. The pedagogical module runs each case by presenting starting information, and then controlling the subsequent presentation of new information to the student. The student module is used by the pedagogical module at various points during a case to analyze the student's answers. As the case progresses, the pedagogical module monitors the student's progress towards specific case goals, such as documentation of findings and diagnoses. Finally, the module evaluates the student's performance.

The pedagogical module uses variants of forward and backward chaining strategies of rules in the knowledge base in order to evaluate student behaviors. For example, a student may document a finding as part of the initial work-up task (which the authors call "search for access rules"). Given the finding, the system then uses forward chaining strategies to consider the rules which have the previously documented finding as a premise. This behavior allows students to receive a valid critique for the work-up of any given end-point, even if they are pursuing a diagnosis which will eventually prove wrong. Another feature provides help if the student makes repeated wrong moves.

Dependent performance measures created by CAI include the amount of information communicated, the number of refuted and accepted premises (rules), and the number of steps in the simulation. The authors state that these various dependent variables can be aggregated into a final score for the entire case. Educational evaluations of the CAI system at Rennes have not yet been published.

PlanAlyzer

The PlanAlyzer was designed by Beck and colleagues at Dartmouth to teach hematologic diseases.[53] It runs on the Macintosh Hypercard platform with a videodisk and television monitor. Students begin a PlanAlyzer case by selecting a case, reviewing an initial patient history, and obtaining additional patient history. At this point the system shows a peripheral smear and provides feedback on the student's interpretation. After viewing the smear (and having corrected faulty interpretations) the student generates a differential diagnosis and a diagnostic plan by choosing from among two dozen hematologic tests. The CDDSS evaluates the student's work-up plan and helps to "prune" unproductive branches by generating normal results for any tests which don't lead to the correct diagnosis. The system also compares the student's strategy with a "gold standard" algorithm for diagnoses present in the knowledge base. At the conclusion of the case, the PlanAlyzer provides a summary of the gold standard work-up and highlights differences between the gold standard and the student's proposed work-up. This summary includes an individualized critique assembled using stock phrases relating to each part of the student work-up.

The PlanAlyzer project was originally intended for use in Dartmouth's innovative sophomore year course, called Scientific Basis of Medicine. From 1988 to 1991 the Dartmouth sophomore classes utilized the system during this course. The PlanAlyzer research team performed two evaluations of the system.[54] The first assessment was a one year (1988) formative evaluation. During this period the prototype text (control) and computer (experimental) cases which covered interpretation of blood smears and electrocardiograms were piloted. The computer and text cases were matched to include the same content, so that training effects could be attributed solely to the computer presentation. The second, summative, evaluation occurred from 1989 to 1990 and was a randomized, controlled, crossover evaluation of the hematologic and cardiology training. Each student trained on the two subject areas, using the computer for one area and text-based instruction for the other. The dependent variables were comparative differences in proficiency and efficiency, as measured on pretests and post-tests, computer data and questionnaire results. Other results included an economic analysis of the PlanAlyzer vs. traditional teaching for the Scientific Basis of Medicine course.

The results showed that the post-test performances of the experimental and control groups, when adjusted for pretest performance in the subject areas, were quite similar. During one year, results were marginally significant in the direction of improved performance for students when they received their anemia training by computer. Students gave favorable reviews to the PlanAlyzer training on evaluation questionnaires. The research team estimated that 96 hours of faculty contact were eliminated by adoption of the PlanAlyzer, and the savings in faculty time could have paid for the Macintosh workstations. Student time also was conserved: 43% less student time was required to complete the material using PlanAlyzer cases as compared to text cases. The Dartmouth faculty were sufficiently satisfied with

PlanAlyzer to make it an ongoing component of the Dartmouth curriculum in 1992. At that time the PlanAlyzer was distributed to 20 other medical schools (including one in Munich) for trial use.

The PlanAlyzer is significant because it was an early example (in the mid-1980s) of a graphical user interface applied to a teaching CDDSS. The PlanAlyzer's developers used the graphical interface in order to overcome clinician and student resistance to tedious operating systems and obscure command syntax. The system was created expressly for student teaching and was not adapted from a general purpose diagnostic system, whereas many other diagnostic systems were primarily intended for decision support. The PlanAlyzer was also unique because it taught a visually-oriented domain, hematologic pathology, which was well suited to the chosen tools. Finally, the PlanAlyzer evaluation studies (unlike those conducted on Iliad) included a completely noncomputer trained group as a control.

NEONATE

NEONATE is a CDDSS which assists nonradiologists in interpreting neonatal chest x-rays.[55] The system was designed by Peter Haug and colleagues for use in the neonatal intensive care unit in Salt Lake's Primary Children's Hospital. NEONATE's knowledge base contains 35 diseases, of which 17 diseases use radiological knowledge frames.

Haug selected ten expert radiologists to create a gold standard list of the x-ray findings and diagnostic statuses of the frames for the 13 chest x-ray films. Each finding was an elemental diagnostic observation on the x-ray (e.g., lower lobe infiltrate). Each diagnostic status was a probability category for the 17 diseases in the knowledge base (e.g., "confirmed," "highly suspected," "pneumonia"). Eighteen pediatric residents at three PGY levels formed the test group. Each resident read the 13 films and each generated a list of findings and diagnostic statuses in the same manner as the expert radiologists. The resident findings were entered manually and NEONATE generated its diagnostic statuses. The agreement was very high between the experts and the computer and the disagreement of experts among themselves was similar to that between experts and the computer.

Haug then evaluated whether NEONATE could improve the residents' x-ray interpretations and subsequent diagnostic judgments. Deviation scores were used to assess the number of diagnosis status disagreements between each practitioner (e.g., each resident, each radiologist) and NEONATE on the set of 13 x-rays. For example, if a resident judged pneumonia to be "confirmed" and NEONATE judged pneumonia to be "unlikely" on case #5, then a disagreement was noted and the deviation score was increased by one for that comparison (two slightly different scores were used, but this was the essential feature of each). The results indicated that NEONATE (using the residents' findings) showed a significantly better agreement with the radiologists' gold standard (mean = 6.637 deviations) than did the average deviation score of the unaided residents (mean = 7.299). When the level of resident training was examined the improvements were significant for the PGY1 and PGY2 residents but not the PGY3 (most senior) trainees.

In summary, the results showed that the CDDSS could potentially improve the accuracy of junior residents when interpreting neonatal chest x-rays. Haug and colleagues did not evaluate whether residents would actually heed NEONATE's recommendations in a practice setting. Also, they did not evaluate whether the residents who gained experience with NEONATE would later improve their performance on chest x-ray diagnosis when they were unaided.

AI/LEARN

AI/Learn is an interactive videodisk system which utilizes the knowledge base of the AI/Rheum CDDSS to teach rheumatology.[34,56] Two teaching strategies are used. The first strategy is to teach visual concepts using exemplar/nonexemplar pairs and immediate feedback. A student might be shown two microscopic images of muscle and asked to pick the one that better demonstrates the finding of myositis. The other strategy uses brief case simulations and delayed feedback. Using this method, the system presents disease profiles which are classical for diagnostic concepts (e.g., myositis) and other profiles which are diagnostic competitors that share some similar features. The student's diagnostic performance on these profiles is reviewed and critiqued, and students may review help modules which provide explanations. The modules contain IF-THEN rules and other teaching slides which are included on the videodisk. While based on the existing AI/Rheum program, additional knowledge engineering was required to prepare the teaching materials. The program was mastered on a videodisk and designed to be controlled by an IBM-PC compatible microcomputer.

LIVER: INFORMATION, EDUCATION AND DIAGNOSIS (LIED)

LIED (Liver: Information, Education and Diagnosis) is a CDDSS for hepatology which was developed at the University of Turin.[57] The system is written in the PROLOG language for IBM-PC compatible computers. LIED provides a diagnostic system, simulated cases, and methods for evaluating the problem solving strategy of users. These LIED functions are similar to those found in Iliad and QMR. LIED contains two parallel knowledge bases for diseases and findings, an inference engine, a case library, and functions which provide the user interface. The classes of diagnostic findings in LIED are classified as "triggers", "necessary findings" and "supplementary findings". The frames are arbitrated by different classes of rules which are called "triggering rules", "early activation rules" and "validation rules". LIED triggers early diagnostic hypotheses and then pursues successive findings which confirm or reject component diagnoses in its differential, thereby simulating the approach of human experts.

LIED provides several educational tools for diagnostic consultations. A tutorial describes LIED's diagnostic algorithm. Another tool is a "system description" module which can analyze LIED's strategy for any specific problem in the case library. This module can describe the evidence supporting the specified condition, the triggering findings for the condition, and the necessary findings which have been instantiated. The module can also display the confirmed rules which support the diagnosis. This module helps users understand how a diagnosis under consideration was evoked and supported. LIED can also select the most useful tests to work-up a differential diagnosis and project the diagnostic impact of proposed tests.

In simulator mode LIED emulates realistic clinical encounters. It introduces each case by means of an initial history and physical examination. The user must respond by providing a list of evoked hypotheses, which LIED evaluates. At this point the user queries LIED for findings to confirm or rule-out the active hypotheses and then revises the hypotheses. The system's response indicates which active hypotheses which are supported and which hypotheses have been confirmed (satisfied a minimum set of rules in the knowledge base). This process of query, hypothesis revision, and hypothesis evaluation is repeated iteratively. Finally, the user must provide a plan for confirming the work-up (e.g., a liver biopsy).

The LIED system has been applied in the educational curriculum at Turin, and the authors are reported to be developing a critiquing mode for the system. This mode would allow students to solve cases and evaluate their work independently.

MYCIN

MYCIN was a pioneering and important CDDSS for infectious disease diagnosis and treatment that was developed by Shortliffe and associates at Stanford University.[58] The system has been extended to include related CDDSS such as ONCOCIN, NEOMYCIN and PUFF.[59] Some of these systems have been evaluated in education, most notably NEOMYCIN and GUIDON.[25]

DISCUSSION

Effectiveness of CDDSS

Many people expect that CDDSS will not be widely accepted in education until clinicians are satisfied that the systems are easy to use and produce accurate results.[60] Unfortunately, few informatics applications have been adequately evaluated in clinical settings.[61] Several groups have recently attempted to correct this deficit. Elstein, Murphy and colleagues assessed the accuracy of Iliad by examining how the diagnostic decisions of students, residents, and attending physicians were affected by use of the system.[44-45] They found that the system functioned midway in accuracy between the residents and the attending physicians. Berner and her colleagues assessed the relative performance of four CDDSS (DXplain, Iliad, Meditel and QMR) and found that the systems performed almost equivalently.[62] Their study found that the proportion of correct diagnoses made by the systems ranged from 0.52 to 0.71 and that each CDDSS suggested about two new relevant diagnoses per case. However, less than half of her experts' diagnoses were contained on the programs' differentials. These results could be condemned as faint praise, but they demonstrate that commercially available, easily disseminated, inexpensive computer programs can begin to approximate the performance of highly trained experts and can equal or surpass resident physicians. Such systems can be invaluable aids for those of us who must sometimes practice (or teach!) "out of our main domains." For these reasons this author uses Iliad and sometimes DXplain to prepare for rounds when he attends on the internal medicine wards.

IMPLEMENTING CDSS IN TEACHING SETTINGS

The University of Utah group to which the author belongs has had extensive experience in implementing the Iliad CDDSS in our medical, nursing, and allied health curricula. We have gained some experience which seems to be reflected by other authors who have done research in this area. The author would like to share five precepts for implementing CDSS in teaching settings.

Use of Informatics Tools to Solve Medical Problems

The first precept is that students should not be taught medical informatics per se, but rather how to solve medical problems using informatics tools. This is a straightforward approach with tremendously high face validity for students who may otherwise be suspicious of "teaching computers for computers sake". Many students will become more interested in informatics details down the road. In fact, this is exactly how many physicians gradually have been lured into the field of medical informatics. Having said that, teachers who adopt CDDSS should take special care to create student exercises which are both relevant and valid. Students will not take well to (or learn from) unnecessarily artificial training measures which lack face validity or introduce unnecessary impediments based on the computer or evaluation technique.[39,60,63] One must create training experiences which have prima facie validity and which also lead to measurable gains in students' knowledge. To achieve these goals the CDDSS must be integrated into the curriculum and used to teach clinically relevant material which is specified in the curriculum.[49-50,60] Implementors should not think that a CDDSS, or any informatics application, will completely replace books or faculty contact in the curriculum. Computers are not an educational panacea. Dr. Homer R. Warner, the leader of our research group, has always strongly emphasized what he calls "the human touch". The human touch includes training the faculty to use the CDDSS together with the students as they jointly explore diagnostic explanations and therapeutic alternatives. It also features comprehensive student training, support, and performance feedback. The faculty's advice and assistance is key to creating a useful CDDSS-assisted curriculum which can take advantage of opportunities for student enrichment and better meet student needs. Consequently, each school and faculty must tailor their CDDSS and informatics implementation to fit unique local conditions and resources.

Faculty Role Models

A second precept is that CDDSS implementors must also increase the informatics knowledge of the faculty and residents. Students have many powerful role models among these clinicians, and imitate them shamelessly. If the students' most important role models don't use the CDDSS, if they don't check their own e-mail, if they have someone else log onto the clinical information system for them, and have a librarian perform all MEDLINE searches, the students will (correctly) conclude that these skills are not important and will not be evaluated (except perhaps by those crazy informaticians in the basement). In evaluation terms, the face validity of the informatics assignments will be low and this will impair the adoption of the system. The faculty must be effectively educated in their own use of CDDSS and informatics technologies, starting with a core group of course directors, small group leaders, and local opinion leaders. When students observe their faculty and residents using a variety of informatics tools, they will naturally seek to use these same tools to locate, validate, manage, and apply medical knowledge to practice.

Protected Curricular Time for Informatics Requirements

A third recommendation is that the CDDSS should be required in the curriculum and that adequate time be allocated to computer activities. If this is not done, students will either feel left out or that they are being unfairly used as computer "guinea pigs". A critical concept is that students do not have time for optional work on the computer. Like their professors, they focus their efforts on activities which are required, evaluated, and rewarded. Therefore, adequate curricular time must be planned to allow students to complete their computer work. At Utah our Clerkship Director frees up the junior students for Iliad training and simulated cases. The underclassmen are similarly freed up for their MEDLINE, Internet, Iliad, electronic mail and other training and computer exercises. To assist them in completing their subsequent computer assignments, they are assigned blocks of time in the form of "open labs" (with faculty preceptors) in the computer classrooms. Students cannot be expected to complete computer assignments that are simply piled on top of an existing curriculum. For this reason informatics innovations must be built into the curriculum through the local equivalent of a Dean's Curriculum Committee. Many schools are now undergoing curricular reforms to incorporate problem-based experiences. These reform-minded times are good opportunities for informaticians and evaluators to "design in" informatics experiences.

Training and Support

A fourth precept is that students assigned to use a CDDSS must receive adequate initial hands-on training and continuing support. The systems cannot be regarded as self teaching. A CDDSS is typically at least as difficult to use as fully featured word processors, and this assessment neglects the content aspects of the comprehensive, detailed medical knowledge base which accompanies a CDDSS, but not a word processor. The author believes the training should ideally take the form of hands-on demonstrations and subsequent practice sessions with feedback. Students must not be placed in the position of having to fulfill required assignments, only to find themselves stymied by lack of adequate preparation to use the assigned tools. The student training should also include some instruction in the basic concepts of decision theory (e.g., Bayes' theorem, decision trees) relevant to the assigned CDDSS, so that students do not regard the system as a mysterious black box. Students are often taught these concepts without any immediate opportunity to apply them, and as a result they are almost universally forgotten. The CDDSS training and subsequent application is a good opportunity to make the concepts more clinically relevant. For example, our Iliad students had a two and one-half hour initial training session, subsequent weekly practice and feedback sessions (Iliad "office hours"), and 24-hour beeper support by an informatics fellow. We provided such comprehensive training and support in order to minimize error variance in our evaluation results. In a nonevaluation setting, or when students and faculty are uniformly "up to speed" on a CDDSS, it is likely that less support would be necessary.

Evaluation

Our fifth precept relates to evaluation. Most CDDSS systems are designed to serve some educational role. However, few have been comprehensively evaluated to determine their educational efficacy. This finding is undoubtedly due to the difficulty and expense of evaluation and to the relative glamour of systems engineering compared to the slogging work of evaluation. All adopters should at least perform a simple evaluation to determine the acceptability of a CDDSS system they have just implemented. A simple evaluation might consist of an implementation description and an assessment of student satisfaction, student perceived learning, and faculty perceived learning. A more comprehensive set of evaluations should be considered if resources such as external funding are available. Many important questions are raised when such an evaluation is designed. The dependent variable must be crisply defined and testing conditions must be controlled, yet valid in an educational setting. We have chosen to exploit the domain specificity of human learning to train all students using the computer, but to train them in different domains. This approach also minimizes student reactivity, as discussed above. Nevertheless a multi-center study might well include some groups that are not trained on the computer, or a school with several curricular pathways might lend itself to a different design. Dependent variables are also key design elements. While the Iliad system was designed to generate and analyze dependent variables, other systems may not do this. One should question the validity of the variables provided by any system or investigator. Ideally, dependent variables should be carefully validated for face, construct, and content validity. Evaluation is not easy; after all, the National Board of Medical Examiners spends millions of dollars creating and validating their examinations. If a comprehensive validation is too difficult or expensive, one should at least try to measure variables that have strong face validity (e.g., diagnostic errors, cost of work-up).

SUMMARY

The computerized diagnostic decision support systems now available are mature enough for targeted adoption in practice and in the curriculum. The systems will continue to be improved and in the future they will be increasingly integrated with clinical documentation systems. Medical curricula are currently being reformulated, and these changes create opportunities to adopt a CDDSS and to evaluate its impact on the medical curriculum.

REFERENCES

1. Masys DR. Medical Informatics: glimpses of the promised land. Acad Med 1989; 64:13-14.
2. Williamson JW, Goldschmit PG, Colton T. The quality of medical literature: an analysis of validation assessments. In: Bailar, JC 3rd,

Mosteller, F, eds. Medical Uses of Statistics. Walton, MA: NEJM Books, 1986:370-391.

3. Schoolman HM. The impact of electronic computers and other technologies on information resources for the physician. Bull N Y Acad Med 1985; 61:283-289.

4. Williamson JW, German PS, Weiss R et al. Health science information management and continuing education of physicians—a survey of U.S. primary care practitioners and their opinion leaders. Ann Intern Med 1989; 110:151-160.

5. Miller RA, Giuse NB. Medical knowledge bases. Acad Med 1991; 66:15-17.

6. Nilasena DS, Lincoln MJ. A computer-generated reminder system improves physician compliance with diabetes preventive care guidelines. Proc Annu Symp Comput Appl Med Care 1995:640-645.

7. Lomas J; Enkin M; Anderson GM et al. Opinion leaders vs. audit and feedback to implement practice guidelines. JAMA 1991; 265:2202-2207.

8. Lomas MA, Anderson GM et al. Do practice guidelines guide practice? The effect of a consensus statement on the practice of physicians. N Engl J Med 1989; 321:1306-1311.

9. Tierney WM, Overhage JM, McDonald CJ. Computerizing guidelines: factors for success. Proc AMIA Fall Symp 1996:459-462.

10. Overhage JM, Tierney WM, McDonald CJ. Computer reminders to implement preventive care guidelines for hospitalized patients. Arch Intern Med 1996; 156:1551-1556.

11. Pestotnik SL, Classen DC, Evans RS et al. Implementing antibiotic practice guidelines through computer-assisted decision support: clinical and financial outcomes. Ann Int Med 1996; 124:884-890.

12. de Dombal FT. Computer-aided diagnosis and decision-making in the acute abdomen. J R Coll Physicians 1975; 9:211-218.

13. Elstein AS, Shulman LS, Sprafka SA. Medical problem solving: an analysis of clinical reasoning. Cambridge, MA: Harvard University Press, 1978.

14. Elstein AS, Shulman LS, Sprafka SA. Medical problem solving: a ten-year retrospective. Eval Health Prof 1990; 13:5-36.

15. Norman GR, Tugwell P, Feightner JW et al. Knowledge and clinical problem-solving ability. Med Educ 1985; 19:344-356.

16. Schmidt HG, Norman GR, Boshuizen HPA. A cognitive perspective on medical expertise: theory and implications. Acad Med 1990; 65:611-621.

17. Fu LS, Huff S, Bouhaddou O et al. Estimating frequency of disease findings from combined hospital databases: a UMLS project. Proc Annu Symp Comput Appl Med Care 1991:373-377.

18. Haug PJ, Gardner RM, Tate KE et al. Decision support in medicine: examples from the HELP system. Comput Biomed Res 1994; 27:396-418.

19. Yu H, Haug PJ, Lincoln MJ, Turner C, Warner HR. Clustered knowledge representation: Increasing the reliability of computerized expert systems. Proc Annu Symp Comput Appl Med Care 1988:126-130.
20. Giuse DA, Giuse NB, Miller RA. A tool for the computer-assisted creation of QMR medical knowledge base disease profiles. Proc Annu Symp Comput Appl Med Care 1991:978-979.
21. Giuse DA, Giuse NB, Miller RA. Consistency enforcement in medical knowledge base construction. Artif Intell Med 1993; 5:245-252.
22. Giuse DA, Giuse NB, Bankowitz RA et al. Heuristic determination of quantitative data for knowledge acquisition in medicine. Comput Biomed Res 1991; 24:261-272.
23. Warner HR. Computer-Assisted Medical Decision Making. New York: Academic Press, 1979.
24. Lincoln MJ, Turner CW, Haug PJ et al. Iliad training enhances medical students' diagnostic skills. J Med Syst 1991; 15:93-109.
25. Shortliffe EH, Perreault LE, eds. Medical Informatics. Reading, MA: Addison Wesley Publishing, 1990.
26. Li YC, Haug PJ, Warner HR. Automated transformation of probabilistic knowledge for a medical diagnostic system. Proc Annu Symp Comput Appl Med Care 1994:765-769.
27. Newell A, Shaw JC, Simon HA. Elements of a theory of human problem solving. Psychol Rev 1958; 65:151-166.
28. Kassirer JP. Diagnostic reasoning. Ann Intern Med 1989; 110:893-900.
29. Barrows HS, Norman GR, Neufeld VR et al. The clinical reasoning of randomly selected physicians in general medical practice. Clin Invest Med 1982; 5:49-55.
30. Kassirer JP, Gorry GA. Clinical problem-solving—a behavioral analysis. Ann Intern Med 1978; 89:245-255.
31. Pople HE Jr. Heuristic methods for imposing structure on ill-structured problems: the structuring of medical diagnostics. In: Szolovits P, ed. Artificial Intelligence in Medicine. AAAS Symposium Series. Boulder, CO: Westview Press, 1982, 119-190.
32. Kassirer JP, Kopelman RI. Cognitive errors in diagnosis: instantiation, classification, and consequences. Am J Med 1989; 86:433-440.
33. Voytovich AE, Rippey RM, Suffredini A. Premature conclusions in diagnostic reasoning. J Med Educ 1985; 60:302-307.
34. Lee AS, Cutts JH, Sharp GC et al. AI/LEARN network. The use of computer-generated graphics to augment the educational utility of a knowledge-based diagnostic system (AI/RHEUM). J Med Syst 1987; 11:349-358.
35. Miller R, Masarie FE, Myers J. Quick Medical Reference (QMR) for diagnostic assistance. MD Comput 1986; 3:34-48.
36. First MB, Soffer LJ, Miller RA. QUICK (Quick Index to Caduceus Knowledge): Using the Internist-I/Caduceus knowledge base as an electronic textbook of medicine. Comput Biomed Res 1985; 18: 137-165.

37. Parker RC, Miller RA. Creation of realistic appearing simulated patient cases using the INTERNIST-1/QMR knowledge base and interrelationship properties of manifestations. Methods Inf Med 1989; 28:346-351.

38. Miller RA, Schaffner KF. The logic of problem-solving in clinical diagnosis: a course for second-year medical students. J Med Educ 1982; 57:63-65.

39. Miller RA, Masarie FE. Use of the Quick Medical Reference (QMR) program as a tool for medical education. Methods Inf Med 1989; 28:340-345.

40. Guo D, Lincoln MJ, Haug PJ et al. Exploring a new best information algorithm for Iliad. Proc Annu Symp Comput Appl Med Care 1991:624-628.

41. Turner CW, Williamson JW, Lincoln MJ et al. The effects of Iliad on medical student problem solving. Proc Annu Symp Comput Appl Med Care 1990:478-482

42. Cundick RM, Turner CW, Lincoln MJ et al. Iliad as a patient case simulator to teach medical problem solving. Proc Annu Symp Comput Appl Med Care 1989:13:902-906.

43. Lincoln MJ, Turner CW, Haug PJ et al. Iliad's role in the generalization of learning across a medical domain. Proc Annu Symp Comput Appl Med Care 1992:174-178.

44. Elstein AS, Friedman CP, Wolf FM et al. Effects of a decision support system on the diagnostic accuracy of users: a preliminary report. JAMIA 1996; 3:422-428.

45. Murphy GC, Friedman CP, Elstein AS. The influence of a decision support system on the differential diagnosis of medical practitioners at three levels of training. Proc AMIA Fall Symp Comput 1996: 219-223.

46. Lange LL, Haak SW, Lincoln MJ et al. Use of Iliad to improve diagnostic performance of nurse practitioner students. J Nurs Educ 1997; 36:36-45.

47. Barnett GO, Cimino JJ, Hupp JA et al. DXplain—an evolving diagnostic decision-support system. JAMA 1987; 258:67-74.

48. Barnett GO, Hoffer EP, Packer MS et al. DXplain—demonstration and discussion of a diagnostic decision support system. Proc Annu Symp Comput Appl Med Care 1992:822.

49. Barnett GO. Information technology and medical education at Harvard Medical School. In: Salamon R, Protti D, Moehr J, eds. Proceedings Medical Informatics & Education International Symposium. Victoria B.C.: International Medical Informatics Association, 1989:3-5.

50. Barnett GO. Information technology and medical education. JAMIA 1995;2:285-291.

51. Frolich MW, Miller PL, Morrow JS. PATHMASTER: modelling differential diagnosis as "dynamic competition" between systematic

analysis and disease-directed deduction. Comput Biomed Res 1990; 23:499-513.

52. Fontaine D, Le Beux P, Riou C et al. An intelligent Computer-Assisted Instruction system for clinical case teaching. Methods Inf Med 1994; 33:433-445.
53. Beck JR, O'Donnell JF, Hirai F et al. Computer-based exercises in anemia diagnosis (PlanAlyzer). Methods Inf Med 1989; 28:364-369.
54. Lyon HC, Healy JC, Bell JR et al. PlanAlyzer, an interactive computer-assisted program to teach clinical problem solving in diagnosing anemia and coronary heart disease. Acad Med 1992; 67:821-828.
55. Franco A, King JD, Farr FL et al. An assessment of the radiological module of NEONATE as an aid in interpreting chest X-ray findings by nonradiologists. J Med Syst 1991; 15:277-286.
56. Mitchell JA, Lee AS, TenBrinkT et al. AI/Learn: an interactive videodisk system for teaching medical concepts and reasoning. J Med Syst 1987; 11:421-429.
57. Console L, Molino G, Ripa di Meana V et al. LIED-Liver: information, education and diagnosis. Methods Inf Med 1989; 31:284-297.
58. Shortliffe EH. Computer-Based Medical Consultations: MYCIN. New York, NY: Elsevier Computer Science Library, Artificial Intelligence Series, 1976.
59. Hickam DH, Shortliffe EH, Bischoff MB et al. The treatment advice of a computer-based cancer chemotherapy protocol advisor. Ann Intern Med 1985; 103:928-936.
60. Siegal JA, Parrino TA. Computerized diagnosis: implications for clinical education. Med Educ 1988; 22:47-54.
61. Lundsgaarde HP. Evaluating medical expert systems. Soc Sci Med 1987; 241:805-819.
62. Berner ES, Webster GD, Shugerman AA et al. Performance of four computer-based diagnostic systems. N Engl J Med 1994; 330:1792-1796.
63. Weed LL. Physicians of the future. N Engl J Med 1981; 304:903-907.

================ CHAPTER 6 ================

Decision Support
for Patients

Holly Brügge Jimison and Paul Phillip Sher

This chapter is designed to introduce the concept of computer-based diagnostic and other decision support systems for patients. It is difficult to separate these systems from the more general area of consumer health informatics. Consumer health informatics represents a diverse field devoted to the development, implementation, and research on telecommunication and computer applications designed to be used by consumers to access information on a wide variety of health care topics. This technology, both hardware and software, is part of a growing trend toward empowering consumers to take a more active role in their own health care and to provide the necessary information to enhance their decision making. Today, more than ever, consumers are using information technology as either a substitute for traditional physician-based medical information or as a supplement to the information provided by health care professionals in the course of clinical encounters.

ROLE OF CONSUMER HEALTH INFORMATICS
IN PATIENT CARE

Research studies have shown that access to health information can enable patients to be more active participants in the treatment process, leading to better medical outcomes.[1-4] Health education is an important aspect of doctor-patient communication. Patients report that they want to be informed about their medical condition,[5-6] and the process of sharing information enhances the doctor-patient relationship. More recently, there has been movement to provide health information via computers. Computer-based information systems for patients have been developed to assist with informed consent,[7] improving coping skills[8-9] and decision-making skills.[8] Involvement in one's medical care also involves the concepts of patient empowerment and self-efficacy.

EMPOWERMENT AND SELF-EFFICACY

Empowerment and self-efficacy are closely linked concepts. In general, empowerment can be thought of as the process that enables people to "own" their own lives and have control over their destiny. It is closely related to health outcomes in that powerlessness has been shown to be a broad-based risk factor for disease. Studies demonstrate that patients who feel "in control" in a medical situation have better outcomes than those who feel "powerless."[10-12]

Similarly, self-efficacy is a patient's level of confidence that he or she can perform a specific task or health behavior in the future. Several clinical studies have shown self-efficacy to be the variable most predictive of improvements in patients' functional status.[13-20] For example, in a study of functional status after bypass surgery, self-efficacy explained more variability in functional status outcomes than did measures of disease severity, functional capacity, comorbidity, or preoperative functioning.[21] Additionally, in a study on patients with rheumatoid arthritis, the degree of perceived self-efficacy was correlated with reduced pain and joint inflammation and improved psychosocial functioning.[15] In cancer patients, a strong positive correlation was found between self-efficacy and quality of life and mood.[22] Perceived self-efficacy was shown to play a significant role in smoking cessation relapse rate, pain management, control of eating and weight, success of recovery from myocardial infarction, and adherence to preventive health programs.[23]

Given the strong influence of empowerment and self-efficacy on health outcomes, it is important to incorporate a focus on these concepts when designing systems for patient use. The feeling of empowerment can be enhanced, for instance, by support groups linked via their computers, which allow patients to feel "connected" to someone else with a similar medical problem. This has been demonstrated by the CHESS (Comprehensive Health Enhancement and Support

System) in women with breast cancer and patients with AIDS.[8,9,24] An important measure of success of health information systems is how well they promote empowerment and self-efficacy for patients.

PATIENT PREFERENCES

As medical care increasingly focuses on chronic disease, it is especially important that patient preferences regarding the long-term effects of their medical care be taken into account. For patients to be adequately informed for making decisions regarding their medical care, it is important that they obtain information about the quality of life associated with the possible medical outcomes of these decisions. Yet, the reliable assessment of a patient's preferences and risk attitudes for clinical outcomes is probably the weakest link in clinical decision making. Recent efforts to explore the use of computers in communication about health outcomes and in assessing patients' preferences for various health outcomes have started to address these issues.[25-27] Information on patient preferences is important for tailoring information to patients and for providing decision support.[25] Tailored information has been found to be more effective in providing consumer information[28] and is preferred by patients.[29] In addition to differences in preferences for health outcomes, patients differ in the degree to which they choose to be involved in decision-making. Research confirms that age (younger), sex (females greater than males) and education level (better educated) are strong predictors of the desire to be involved in medical decisions. There is also a higher desire to be involved in medical decisions that appear to require less medical expertise, such as a knee injury as opposed to a cancerous growth.[29]

THE COMPUTER AS A HEALTH INFORMATION MEDIUM

There has been an increase in research devoted to testing the effectiveness of various formats and types of media for conveying health information to consumers.[30-34] These studies tend to show that video and slides are educationally more effective than books and audiotapes. Computer approaches have the additional advantages of interactivity, providing feedback in the learning process, and the ability to tailor information to the individual patient. However, in many cases, more research is required to demonstrate the effectiveness of computer approaches. In addition, designers of systems for patients have not always been sufficiently sensitive to human-computer

---

Table 6.1. Design guidelines for a consumer health information system

---

Intuitive Interface
- Graphical metaphors easily understood by the general populace
- Designed for use by naive, untrained users
- On-line help available at every stage
- Immediate word definitions available in every application

Complete Coverage / Coordination
- Single location for information on diseases and health concerns
- Coordinated with routine medical care

Hierarchical Presentation
- Simple summary information presented first
- More detail and complexity available as desired
- Guided movement through databases
- User requests anticipated, pre-search to improve speed

Presentation Tailored to the Individual
- Material presented appropriate for the assessed reading level
- Material presented appropriate for education and medical expertise
- Material presented in a culturally sensitive manner
- Material presented in the appropriate language
- Material tailored to history and assessed patient-specific health risks
- Patient preferences incorporated

Facilitate Quality Decision Making
- Health outcomes information included
- Patient preferences on health outcomes incorporated
- Summary of tailored decision support information

Option for Printout
- Ability for the patient to have material to take home / share with family
  included

---

interface issues. The design of a system for general health education for patients requires specifications that meet a variety of needs. Table 6.1 outlines the design guidelines for a consumer health information system.

TECHNOLOGY FOR PATIENT DECISION SUPPORT SYSTEMS

Advances in computer technology and communications have provided consumers with access to enormous amounts of information. From its earliest beginnings in the 1970s, personal computers have become a ubiquitous part of the workplace and of many homes. It is estimated that there are about 25 million home computers and the number is steadily growing. The power of today's systems has expanded access to information dramatically. From 1996 to 1998, the most popular-priced personal computer ($1000-$2000), will change from a processor with three million circuits to one with six million circuits. Presently, processor speeds range from 120-200 MHz. By 1998, processor speeds will range from 300-450 MHz. Technological developments impact the way information is stored and displayed. The trend today is to merge text, images, audio, video, graphics, and animation into an integrated multimedia program. In the future, the personal computer may be supplanted by such technologies as cable modems and WebTV which will turn televisions into new information tools. Some of the technologies that enhance the dissemination of health information are briefly discussed in the following sections.

Videodisc

Videodisc systems are widely used for interactive teaching programs. These devices can store video, as well as still frames, and offer rapid searching, freeze-frame and slow motion. Systems are available as stand-alones that do not require a separate computer, as well as more advanced models that link directly with microcomputer control. This technology has been used successfully for education and training. The Foundation for Shared Decision Making has developed several interactive videodiscs to assist patients in participating in their treatment decisions. One of their first systems was designed to inform men with enlarged prostates about issues associated with choosing surgical treatment or "watchful waiting."[35] They have also developed similar systems for breast cancer, ischemic heart disease, low back pain, and hypertension. These systems use patient-specific information (age, sex, symptoms, medical history, test results) to calculate patient-specific probabilities for treatment outcomes. The videodiscs contain interviews with patients who have undergone various treatment options to provide system users with a better understanding of potential health outcomes.

Compact Disc (CD-ROM)

First introduced as audio discs (CDs), CD-ROM technology led the multimedia revolution. Presently, CD-ROM (Compact Disc—Read Only Memory), CD-I (Compact Disc—Interactive), and PhotoCD are used in a wide variety of multimedia health programs and also serve as the storage media for databases and textbook references. CD-ROMs have a capacity of 600 megabytes (300,000 text pages). Philips and Sony have jointly developed a high-density CD-ROM called DVD (Digital Video Disc) with a capacity of 3.7 Gigabytes, more than five times the capacity of today's discs. In the future, this capacity could increase to 7.4 Gigabytes with two readable layers. Most of the home references and library databases use this storage media. In the future, one DVD disc could represent a personal library of information that could be accessed at home or over a single disk server.

Compact Disc Interactive (CD-I)

CD-I is a technology developed by Philips and Sony that combines audio, video, and text in a single player that can be used on a standard television. It has been used successfully for home entertainment, as well as for home education, information and training. Examples of consumer health products that utilize CD-I include InfoTouch Health Kiosk (Novare International), Breast Self-Examination and Carpal Tunnel Syndrome (MED.I.A. Inc.). InfoTouch Health Kiosk consists of 20 video and slide shows which are designed to provide basic health information, treatment for simple medical problems and when to consult a physician. The kiosks are installed in Kroger Drug Stores in Texas. Breast Self-Examination uses multimedia visuals to present the latest American Cancer Society guidelines for breast self-examination. Carpal Tunnel Syndrome uses animation and text to provide patients with an overview of Carpal Tunnel Syndrome including anatomy, signs and symptoms, diagnostic tests, and treatment. In addition to home use, CD-I is very useful in the physician's office and waiting room.

Internet and World-Wide Web (WWW)

In 1969, The Department of Defense's Advanced Research Projects Agency created the Internet's predecessor, DARPANET, which linked mainframe computers at four geographically distant sites. It became ARPANET in 1972 and consisted of 40 computers networked to facilitate communication among researchers. The National Science Foundation assumed control of the network infrastructure in 1987 and expanded access. Today, this rudimentary network has grown to become the vast interconnections of the Internet with an estimated 30 million computer users. The exact number of sites and users is not known and the statistics on use vary considerably, but have shown a steady increase (see URL-http://nw.com for the latest statistics).

The recent dramatic expansion of the Internet has been through the World-Wide Web (WWW or Web), first developed by CERN (European Centre for Particle Physics). The WWW supports multimedia through a graphical interface that allows sophisticated text formatting, graphics and embedded hypertext links to other locations on the Web. The Web contains vast amounts of consumer health and medical information. Much of this information is posted by government agencies, medical foundations, universities, medical schools, individual physicians, health insurance companies, and health care providers, special interest support groups and many health and medical-related companies (pharmaceutical industry, medical supplies, etc.). There is also health information, or links to sites with health information, on individuals' personal Web pages. At present, the WWW is a democracy of free information exchange without regard for accuracy or objectivity. "Viewer beware" is the caveat for anyone looking for medical information on the Internet.[36] Some attempts have been made to rate and to evaluate sites. The American Medical Informatics Association (AMIA) Internet Working Group developed Medical Matrix, which includes links to a variety of health informatics sites. The working group developed criteria to describe and evaluate information resources and is attempting to formalize the review process (personal communication, Gary Malet, DO). John Renner, M.D. (Consumer Health Information Research Institute, Independence, MO) maintains a Web site that examines the quality of Internet health information. The site and his weekly column under Internet Health Watch are on the Reuters Health Information Services site (URL-http://www.reutershealth.com). The Appendix to this book contains a list of several useful and interesting Web sites for consumer health information. In addition to Web sites such as these, the major commercial online vendors (America Online, Compuserve, Prodigy) provide access to health information services including the traditional reference materials, databases, as well as support groups and forum discussions of health-related topics. These services also provide forums, chat groups and access to health-related newsgroups.

Community health networks and online self-help networks are becoming more available to consumers, who are being transformed from passive receivers of health care to active participants. AARP Online (American Association of Retired Persons) provides information and forums, for persons aged 50 and older, on a wide range of issues, as well as information on AARP. Coolware World Wide Server-Health Information (Coolware, Inc.) helps people take advantage of the information available on the Internet. One category of health care information provided is in areas such as prevention and alternative medicine. CANCERNET is a quick and easy way to obtain cancer information from the National Cancer Institute (NCI) using electronic mail.[37] CANCERNET offers patient information statements from the NCI's Physician Data Query (PDQ) database, fact sheets on various cancer topics from the NCI's Office of Cancer Communications, and citations and abstracts on selected topics from the CANCERLIT database. Selected information is also available in Spanish.

There are many other Internet services: electronic mail, mailing lists, File Transfer Protocol (FTP), Listservers, USENET newsgroups, Telnet and IRC (Internet Relay Chat). Some of these services have wide application in consumer health informatics. Electronic mail and mailing lists allow patients to communicate with each other, as well as with some health care providers. Mailing lists allow groups of people to receive e-mail messages. Listservers are systems dedicated to a particular topic with specialized software to maintain subscription lists and handle e-mail traffic. There are numerous health-related Listservers, such as ALZHEIMER (Alzheimer's Disease), ALT-MED-RES (alternative medicine research), CANCER-L (public list for cancer-related issues), CAREPL-L (database of archived care plans), and FIROM-L (Fibromyalgia). USENET newsgroups provide a more informal approach to communications. There are many medical and health-related newsgroups among the over 4800 newsgroups on the Usenet (User's Network). The activity varies, but all messages to the newsgroup are available to anyone who accesses the newsgroup. Examples of such medical newsgroups include misc.health.diabetes, alt.support.diabetes.kids, alt.support.depression, alt.support.diet, and alt.support.menopause. Many of these groups provide support to patients suffering from particular diseases. Patients find that communicating with other patients is very helpful, and this communication can actually improve health outcomes.[8] Before the development of the newsgroups, bulletin boards (BBSs) were the main mechanism for group communication on specialized topics. There are 60,000 bulletin boards covering diverse subjects including health care, special interest and support groups. IRC is a multi-user chat computer protocol that allows the computer connection of users and provides a means for interactive disease-oriented support-group communication. Listservers, newsgroups and BBSs all provide a mechanism for users to communicate with each other about any and all aspects of health care. Most of these resources are unmoderated; therefore all information needs to be verified. In chronic diseases, the newsgroups provide an important social function by allowing patients to share experiences about their disease, treatment and prognosis. In fact, the entire function of some newsgroups is to provide such support.

Cable Modem

As the Internet grows in complexity and includes more multimedia elements, access time becomes an important consideration. A cable modem is a modem that is connected to the network interface card of a computer using a cable television network line. Cable modem technology is 100 times faster than a 14.4 standard modem, 50 times faster than the newer 28.8 modems and 12 times faster than an ISDN line. Cable modems will allow Internet users to download text, video, audio and animation at sufficiently high speed to make them usable. Cable companies may install CD-ROM servers and charge for access to many of the programs that are mentioned in this chapter. Implementation has been slow and pricing is very geographically dependent. Modem and installation will cost approximately $100 and monthly charges will run around $50. More information on cable modem technology can be found on the Internet. A cable modem resource site is at http://rpcp.mit.edu/~gingold/cable/.

Phone services are available to provide prerecorded health information on a wide variety of health-related subjects for those not equipped with a computer. This service is usually purchased by hospitals or libraries as a service to their customers.

WebTV

The Web TV technology developed by Sony and Philips consists of a TV set-top box (or built-in) which connects to the TV and a telephone line. The box will cost approximately $350 with a monthly charge for unlimited Internet access of about $20. This charge also includes e-mail service. Either the remote control or a separate keyboard will allow the user to navigate the Internet. There is tremendous potential for this technology to provide health information to millions of households without personal computers.

CONVERGING TECHNOLOGIES IN THE FUTURE

The present trend in both computer and telecommunication hardware and software is to merge all communications technologies together. The home television of the future will likely contain a computer, FAX, telephone communication, video conferencing capabilities and high speed cable modem connections. Consumers will have the capability to communicate interactively not only to acquire health information, but also to consult with health care professionals (telemedicine). The convergence of these digital technologies "will be key to a superior coordination and collaboration among providers, agencies, caregivers and families to integrate medical, health, mental health, social and economic support services."[38]

DIAGNOSTIC AND OTHER DECISION SUPPORT SYSTEMS FOR PATIENTS

The number of commercial computer products to support patients' health information needs is expanding so rapidly that it is difficult to maintain an updated inventory. The Informed Patient Decisions Group at Oregon Health Sciences University created a directory of these products.[39] At the time of publication, there were well over six hundred software products covering the spectrum of consumer health information needs including such diverse areas as patient education, health promotion and prevention, nutrition and fitness, self-triage, maintaining health records, decision-making and health reference libraries.[40]

The primary focus for the remainder of this chapter will be on systems that provide diagnostic and other types of decision support for patients. The general health references that provide decision support will briefly be reviewed. There are few commercial systems that can truly be called diagnostic systems, i.e., those systems that aid a patient in making a diagnosis based on the input of medically-related information, usually symptoms. Those systems that do perform this function will be discussed in greater detail.

A number of products are available as general home health care references. These are designed as a single source of general health information similar to the home health references found with encyclopedias or as textbooks. The software is CD-ROM-based and available for either Macintosh™ or Windows™ based systems. The programs have some type of search engine (for subject search), as well as the ability to print information. These products can be divided into those that are typically used by consumers at home with personal computers and the larger, more costly databases that are usually seen in health reference libraries.

HOME REFERENCES

In general, these products are health reference encyclopedias that, in most cases, were produced initially as textbooks and subsequently converted to electronic media. One such program for home use is the Mayo Clinic Family Healthbook™ (IVI Publishing). Although mainly text, it also includes 75 videos, 600 photos and illustrations, and audio narration with information on over 1,000 medical conditions and 3,000 drugs. The program includes a Web browser and automatic link to their Mayo Clinic site (http://www.mayo.ivi.com). Medical HouseCall™ and Pediatric HouseCall™ (Applied Medical Informatics, now published by Mosby Consumer Health) are family medical software packages that encompass symptom analysis, a pharmacy guide, a family medical records maintenance module, and a 5,000 page medical encyclopedia. The Family Doctor™ (Creative Multimedia) contains a library of health information resources, as well as first aid information. The AMA Family Medical Guide™ (American Medical Association and Dorling Kindersley Ltd.) is designed to provide comprehensive health information and includes sections on first aid, drugs and common medical conditions. It contains 900 photos and illustrations and 60 videos and animations. Similarly, Dr. Schueler's Home Medical Advisor Pro™ (Dr. Schueler's Health Informatics, Inc., now published by The Learning Company) is a three CD-ROM set that integrates video, sound, and images into a comprehensive health reference with over 2,000 photographic images and sounds and an extensive library of full motion video clips (two hours). The program teaches about health, analyzes drug interactions, produces medico-legal documents and assists in keeping detailed personal medical records.

Four of these products (Medical HouseCall™, Pediatric HouseCall,™ Dr. Schueler's Home Medical Advisor Pro™ and the AMA Family Medical Guide™) have the capability to perform diagnostic decision support and will be discussed in greater detail later in this chapter.

LIBRARY REFERENCE DATABASES

Health resource libraries often subscribe to larger databases that are too costly for the average consumer. These databases collect information from journals, newspapers, and other media into a single source. The Health Reference Center™ (Information Access Company) is a database with three years of medical information from periodicals, pamphlets, and reference books. Over 150 titles are indexed, with full text coverage of 100 titles, full text of over 500 medical information pamphlets, and indexing and full text of five leading medical reference books. The abstracts of technical articles are written in lay language. Recent versions also include patient education handouts from Clinical Reference Systems. This database can be accessed via the Web or CD-ROM. Similarly, MDX Health Digest™ (CD Plus) is another large health reference database that indexes consumer newspapers and magazines, as well as standard medical journals. The database includes bibliographic citations from over 200 publications, journals, newspapers, and newsletters from 1988 to the present. Detailed abstracts are written by health care professionals in easily understood language. Finally, HealthSource™ (EBSCO Publishing) is a health reference database that provides access to indexing and abstracts for nearly 200 publications concerning diet and nutrition, exercise, medical self-care, drugs and alcohol, consumer issues, aging, family safety and health. HealthSource journals have been selected by analysis of health-related titles with the highest subscriber volume from both academic and large public libraries. The program offers key word searches, full text of articles, including charts and graphs, for 57 journals, and 500 health-related pamphlets.

Symptoms, Diseases, Diagnoses, Diagnostic Procedures, Treatments

This category contains a diverse collection of software products that enumerate disease signs and symptoms, as well as explanations for diagnostic tests and treatment options. An example of such a program is Complete Guide to Symptoms and Illness™ (Great Bear Technology), a resource with information on causes, diagnoses, treatments, complications, and outcomes of hundreds of medical problems. The software includes detailed multimedia-based material on more than 800 symptoms, over 500 illnesses, and 177 surgical procedures, as well as suggestions on how individuals can live longer and stay healthier. Specialized programs have been produced to cover high interest topics, such as Breast Cancer Lighthouse (Gold Standard Media), a breast cancer resource that includes 30 minutes of audio quotes from 14 breast cancer survivors.

Drug Information

There are several drug reference programs designed to help consumers with information on prescription and nonprescription medications, including drug interactions and side effects. One such program is Mayo Clinic Family Pharmacist™ (IVI Publishing). The program enables users to obtain nontechnical information on over 8,000 brand, generic and over-the-counter drugs. The program also provides online access for answers to questions, such as why a drug is prescribed; dosage and usage information; adverse reactions; warnings; precautions; and possible interactions with other drugs, foods, and beverages. The major home health reference software programs listed above contain drug modules that perform similar functions.

Patient Advice and Handouts

Patients and physicians often agree that the doctor is the most appropriate source of medical information,[41-42] but there can be misunderstandings when only oral information is provided.[43] Several options exist for supplementing physicians' advice. Written information that physicians give to patients has traditionally been provided in the form of one-page handouts or brochures on specific topics of interest. Kahn reviewed programs for computer generated patient handouts.[44] An example of this type of program is Health Advisor™ (Clinical Reference Systems, Ltd.), that generates patient advice handouts on over four hundred medical and surgical topics. Exit-Writer (Parker-Hill Associates) contains a database of 300 choices from such categories as medications and treatments, diagnosis and miscellaneous items. CareNotes (Micromedex) contains a similar database, including a detailed drug information module called DrugNotes. Selected patient handouts are also available on the World-Wide Web (see Appendix).

EMERGENCY FIRST AID

Programs are available to teach first aid and to give home emergency medical advice. Although emergency medical information is available in the general home health references listed previously, some programs are designed specifically for this information. For example, First Aid Tutorial™ (Marketing Services Corporation of America) presents basic first aid treatment for common medical emergencies including bleeding, shock, fractures, burns and poisoning.

SELF-HELP AND PREVENTION

Dr. Schueler's Self Health™ is designed as a personal health manager with modules that help users learn about disease risk, perform health evaluations, maintain medical records, estimate health care costs and manage health expenses. The program contains 70 minutes of video clips, as well as the capability to create 3D graphs to monitor progress toward health goals. An interesting feature of this program is a cost analysis section that provides information on costs for procedures by geographic area. Other specialized programs are available to help selected preventive health areas. One example is LifeSign™ (PICS, Inc.), a smoking cessation program implemented by a credit card-sized computer. During the first seven days of the program, users simply press a button each time they smoke. LifeSign™ then uses this information to tailor a gradual withdrawal program based on each smoker's habit. During the withdrawal phase (10-28 days, depending on habit), LifeSign™ prompts users on when to smoke and gradually increases the intervals between cigarettes. Because smokers cut down slowly, severe cravings and withdrawal symptoms are avoided. The complete program includes computer, program guide, motivational video and access to a toll-free help line.

Self-care has an important element of decision-making for patients, in that whenever a symptom or set of symptoms occur, the patient needs to decide whether or not to seek professional medical care or manage the problem at home. Several computer systems have targeted this need. For example, the HealthyLife Self Care Video & Guide™(American Institute for Preventive Medicine) advises patients on self-triage using a flow-chart format, linking to materials on self-care procedures. Similarly, the AMA Family Medical Guide uses flow-charts and branching algorithms to instruct patients on when to see a doctor and when to administer self-care (further described in the section on Diagnostic Decision Support). Finally, the Healthwise Knowledgebase contains both a Symptom Manager, with advice on self care and when to see a doctor, as well as a Disease Manager, with information on treatment options for shared decision making.

PREPARATION FOR OFFICE VISITS/HISTORY TAKING/HEALTH RECORDS

Preparing in advance for medical appointments can play an important role in effective physician-patient communication and shared decision making. Some of the general health reference programs have modules to help maintain medical records. Computer programs can help patients by organizing information, educating consumers, and keeping a record of important issues that need to be addressed during the encounter. Medical Records™ (Dr. Schueler's Health Informatics, Inc., now published by The Learning Company) allows a user to maintain comprehensive medical records, analyzes over 2,400 drugs for reactions, and prints medico-legal documents. Medical Matters™ (Parsons Technology) helps to monitor medical visits and the costs and insurance activities associated with those visits. It also includes an online copy of the *Random House Health and Medicine Dictionary*, a guide to over 5,000 drugs, a listing of over 500 health and medical agencies across the country, and three Medicare references.

DIAGNOSTIC DECISION SUPPORT

In this section of the chapter, we will review computer-based systems that specifically target diagnostic decision support for patients.

MEDICAL HOUSECALL™ AND PEDIATRIC HOUSECALL™

The system design for Medical HouseCall™ and Pediatric HouseCall™ was derived from a diagnostic and treatment expert system for physicians, known as Iliad™ (see chapter 5 for more information on Iliad). The knowledge base and inference engine were

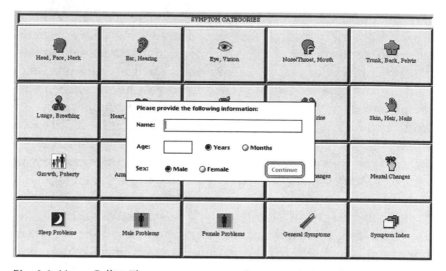

Fig. 6.1. HouseCall™. The program prompts for age and sex and provides a series of body part icons for symptom localization. Reproduced from the CD-ROM, Pediatric HouseCall, originally published by Applied Medical Informatics, with permission from Mosby-Year Book, © 1997.

restructured to accommodate consumer queries and answers.[45-46] The symptom analysis module requires the input of the patient's age and gender. The pediatric software allows entry of age in either years or months. A menu of body parts icons allows the user to enter symptoms (Fig. 6.1). The user also answers a series of YES/NO questions (Fig. 6.2). When this first series of questions is finished, the user can either go back to the symptom categories or click the "Ask Follow-up Questions" button for further questions related to the initial responses. The questions that appear lead to a ranked order of likelihood of diseases based on the symptoms. The probabilities are Bayesian statistical calculations using the Iliad™ program with modifications described below. The user has several options at this point—the program can: (1) show questions the doctor might ask; (2) show less likely causes, which expands the original list to include rare diseases; or (3) print a report. At any time, the user can click on the diseases listed for further information including an explanation of the symptoms, which lists those patient symptoms that are explained by the particular disease and those symptoms that need another explanation.

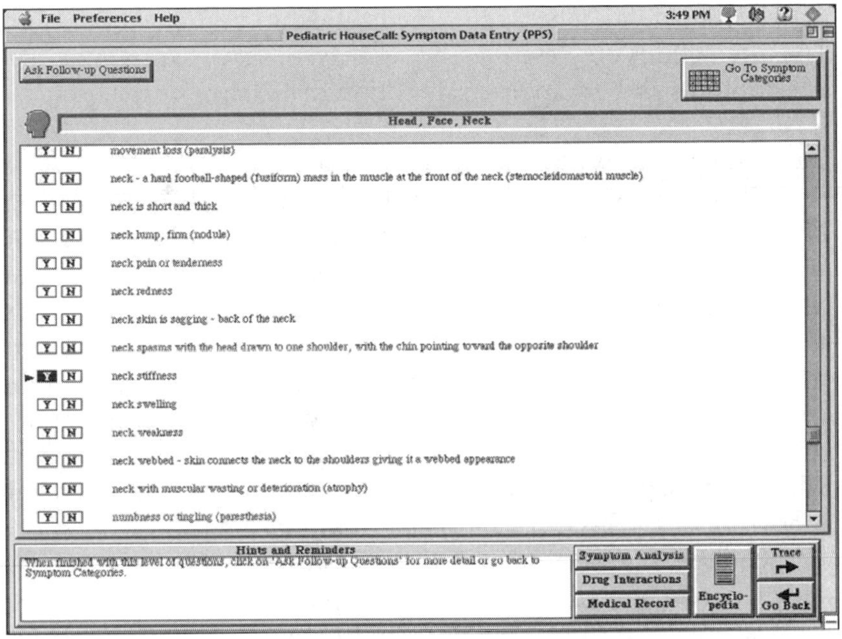

Fig. 6.2. HouseCall™. A list of signs and symptoms is presented for each body location with option to answer YES or NO. Reproduced from the CD-ROM, Pediatric HouseCall, originally published by Applied Medical Informatics, with permission from Mosby-Year Book, ©1997.

The software is careful to point out that the list is not a list of "diagnoses," since a diagnosis list would require physical examination and possible tests. The adaptation of the Iliad™ diagnostic module (knowledge base and inference engine) required some modifications. Physical exam findings and lab tests were eliminated from the knowledge base. The vocabulary was translated into "consumer language." The diagnostic probabilities were adjusted not to exceed 70%, the estimated contribution of historical information to making a diagnosis.[47] Finally, the list combines diseases for cases in which laboratory or physical findings were needed to make the diagnosis.

Another decision support module of the programs is the drug interaction section. The program can advise the user about potential drug interactions of many prescription and over-the-counter drugs, as well as interaction between a medication and caffeine or alcohol. The interactions are described by severity, onset of symptoms, type of symptoms and the appropriate action to be taken by the user.

DR. SCHUELER'S HOME MEDICAL ADVISOR PRO™

There are two decision support components in Home Medical Advisor Pro™, a symptom analysis program for single symptoms and a Symptom Complex Analysis program for multiple symptoms. The single symptom analysis program allows the user to get information about the particular symptom, including possible causes. Users are asked a series of questions to provide further characterization of the symptom. These questions were developed through detailed protocols and flow chart algorithms by physician consultants (Stephen J. Schueler, MD, personal communication). The questions are asked in a series of video clips with a physician asking some of the questions that require a yes/no response. Other questions appear with graphics designed to aid in understanding the symptom and question. Answering this series of yes/no questions leads to a possible cause and associated information window about the disease or cause of the symptom.

The second decision support component of Home Medical Advisor Pro™ is called Symptom Complex Analysis. The Symptom Complex Analysis program starts with a window listing broad categories of symptoms (general; psychological; neurological; skin and nails; eyes; ear, nose and throat; head and neck; chest and breasts; etc.). Each of these categories includes specific symptoms. The user can select as many symptoms as needed (Fig. 6.3). When complete, an analysis button is clicked and a list of possible diagnoses appears in a separate window. The program uses rule-based algorithms to identify diseases that match the symptoms and then restructures the list based on their likelihood. (Stephen J. Schueler, MD, personal communication). The analysis lists possible diseases, categorized in two ways. First, the number of symptoms that match with a particular disease are listed starting with diseases with the most matches. Second, the likelihood probabilities appear in parentheses following the diagnosis and are expressed as very common, common, rare, and very rare. The "diagnoses," like those presented by Medical HouseCall™ and Pediatric HouseCall™, are based only on a patient's observed data and not diagnostic tests.

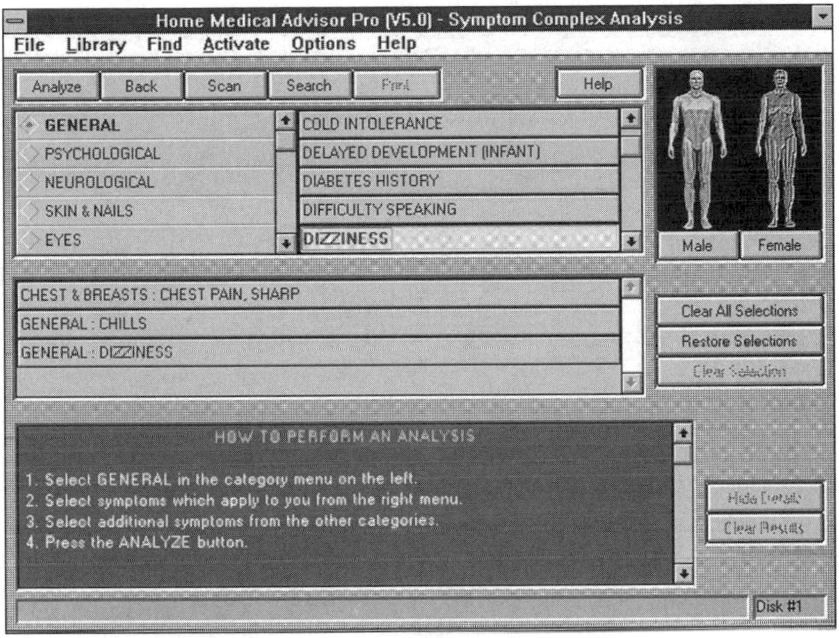

Fig. 6.3. Home Medical Advisor Pro™. The user chooses among the list of symptoms. Each symptom is added to the list. Reproduced from the CD-ROM, Home Medical Advisor Pro, version 5.0, with permission from Dr. Schueler's Health Informatics, Inc. ©1993-1996, all rights reserved.

Home Medical Advisor Pro™ contains a drug interactions module called InteRact. Medication history can either be obtained from the medical records module of this program or the user can enter drugs from a list that includes medications, nicotine, caffeine, alcohol, or foods (Fig. 6.4). When the user asks for an analysis, a list of possible interactions appears in a window below the drug list. The program database contains 500,000 interactions. The company has a Web site for downloading updates, but no demonstration software (URL http://www.drschueler.com). Home Medical Advisor published by The Learning Company (http:store.learningco.com/version.html).

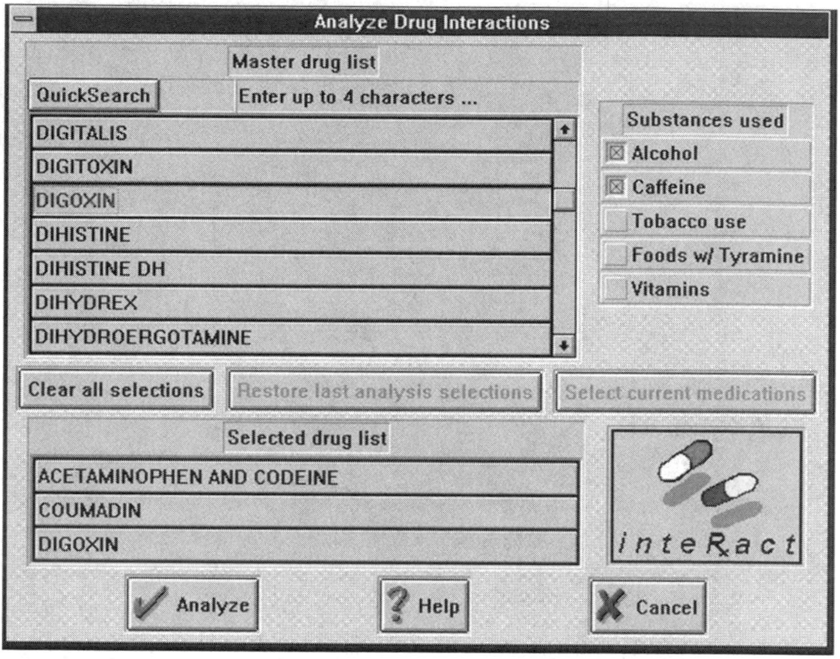

Fig. 6.4. Home Medical Advisor™. The medication module allows the user to enter both drugs as well as substances that are used such as alcohol. Reproduced from the CD-ROM, Home Medical Advisor PRO, version 5.0 with permission from Dr. Schueler's Health Informatics, Inc. © 1993-1996, all rights reserved.

AMA FAMILY MEDICAL GUIDE

The AMA Family Medical Guide is the CD-ROM-based version of the American Medical Association Family Medical Guide published by Random House, Inc. The program consists of seven modules: (1) diseases, disorders and other problems; (2) atlas of the body; (3) symptoms and self-diagnosis; (4) your healthy body; (5) injuries and emergencies; (6) diagnostic imaging techniques; and (7) caring for the sick. The program's diagnostic decision support for men, woman and children consists of 99 symptom flow charts that are organized alphabetically or can be accessed by either pain-site diagrams or body system diagnosis (Fig. 6.5). The diagnostic symptoms charts are flow diagrams in which each question is read to the user by the computer. A "yes" or "no" answer to the question directs the user

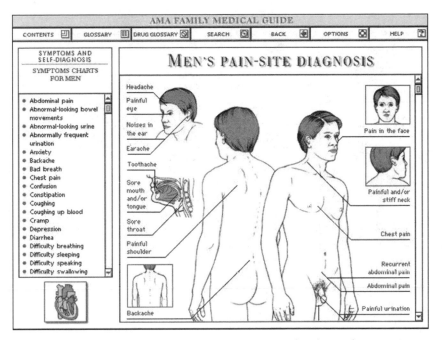

Fig. 6.5. AMA Family Medical Guide™. Symptoms can be chosen from a pain-site chart. Reproduced from Family Medical Guide, CD-ROM, © 1995 American Medical Association, with permission.

through the flow diagram to the next question (Fig. 6.6). If an emergency condition is reached in the flow chart, a red bold message reading "EMERGENCY Get medical help now" appears along with a telephone icon. The message also explains why it may be an emergency with references to the encyclopedia for more information. The company that produces this multimedia software has a Web site at http://www.dk.com.

PATIENT ACCESS TO DIAGNOSTIC DECISION SUPPORT SYSTEMS

As the demand for more health information and decision support grows, the need for wider availability of these systems becomes even more important. Today, these systems can be found in a variety

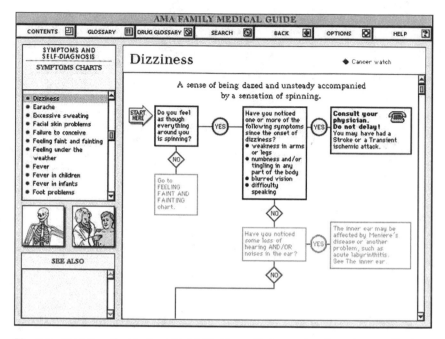

Fig. 6.6. AMA Family Medical Guide™. The self-diagnosing flowcharts will allow the user to answer YES/NO questions and proceed through to a diagnosis or notice to consult a physician. Only the branches that follow the YES/NO answers are highlighted. Reproduced from Family Medical Guide, CD-ROM, © 1995 American Medical Association, with permission.

of settings and in a variety of forms. The most common locations to access these systems are physician waiting rooms, hospitals and health resource libraries, public libraries, worksites, schools, community centers, and, of course, on personal computers in the home. Different systems may require quite different physical locations. For instance, many patients are uncomfortable exploring sensitive health information in a public space.

There are many factors that influence the health information seeking behavior of patients. As documented by Harris, these factors include demographic divisions such as age, gender, disability, race and ethnicity, and socioeconomic status.[48] Research indicates that these demographic variables can predict differences in the amount and type of information about their health that patients want. While some patients do not seek much information, even when the patient desires information, serious barriers still exist to the use of these systems.

A lack of reading ability is a functional barrier affecting use of the systems. Approximately one out of five Americans is functionally illiterate, reading at or below the fifth grade level. Most studies on the comprehension of health education handouts typically show that only half of the patients are able to comprehend written health materials.[49-51] Studies confirmed that patients' reading levels were well below what was needed to understand standard health brochures.[52] In developing health information for patients, one cannot assume that a patient who has completed a certain grade level in school can read at the corresponding level. Numerous studies on literacy and readability confirm the widespread problem of low literacy skills.[53-55] Health materials should be written at least three grade levels lower than the average educational level of the target population.[56] Text characteristics also play an important role in comprehension and retention of material. Organization and clarity need to be considered in creating education materials.[57] Computers with multimedia techniques can serve to correct some of these problems by conveying information through video, audio and graphics that would normally be written text. These systems can also be adapted for multiple foreign languages.

In addition to language and literacy issues, an area that is often overlooked are the cultural issues associated with health information seeking behavior and the willingness to use computers to access health information. Most developers have not invested the time to develop systems that are culturally and linguistically relevant to diverse populations.

Finally, the question of who will pay for the access and use of technologies for consumer health information is still an unresolved issue. Educational and socioeconomic factors still determine access to computers and information technologies. Younger, more affluent, and well educated patients are more likely to have access to home computers, diagnostic software, and the Internet. Older, less affluent, and less well educated patients usually have access only to local public libraries and television. The poor and socioeconomically disadvantaged already have worse health outcomes and worse access to medical care. Special effort is required to ensure ease of access and ease of use of health information systems, so as to not further disadvantage the very people who have the greatest need for these resources.

THE FUTURE OF DIAGNOSTIC DECISION SUPPORT SYSTEMS FOR PATIENTS

Advances in communications and information processing technology will certainly change the way in which medicine is practiced, and will also change the way in which patients receive information and interact with the medical care system. The future holds great promise for consumers becoming empowered participants and assuming a more active role in their medical care decisions through increased and more effective access to health care information. The developers of commercial systems have pushed the field of consumer health informatics forward with many innovative systems. However, to achieve significant improvements in quality of care and health outcomes, researchers and system developers need to focus on bringing the knowledge gained from previous work in health education into the design of new systems. The goals of research on these systems is to develop sound principles to inform the design of new systems for patient use and to measure the benefits derived from the use of those systems. This is a new and rapidly developing field, with significant innovations in the commercial sector. However, research in several areas is needed to move the field forward in providing real benefits to patients' health outcomes and in showing the effectiveness of the systems to purchasers of health care. The criteria for evaluating computer-based diagnostic systems for patients are similar to the criteria for physician systems, namely accuracy and effectiveness.[58] However, the rapid deployment of these systems in an ever changing medical care environment makes critical evaluation of consumer health information systems extremely difficult. Web sites change daily, and access to one system usually means increased access to many others. It is important to understand the potential effectiveness of investments in this area. Careful needs assessment before system development, usability testing during development, controlled clinical trials, and studies of use and outcomes in natural settings are all critical to our understanding of how best to provide health information and decision assistance to patients.

In the final analysis, achieving universal access to health care for all may be accomplished by linking patients to the health care system via the new information technology. Networked health information has great potential for all participants and receivers of health care. Since the vast majority of health-related decisions are made outside of the medical setting,[59] consumer health information resources that include decision support systems for patients can play an important role and may prove to be a cost-effective way to enhance access to health care for the disadvantaged and underserved in our population. It is important to remember, however, that consumers in need of specific health information still depend on health care professionals (doctors, nurses) and their own health care provider. These systems and information resources are important tools to enhance understanding, communication, and, ultimately, health outcomes.

REFERENCES

1. Brody DS, Miller SM, Lerman CE et al. Patient perception of involvement in medical care: relationship to illness attitudes and outcomes. J Gen Intern Med 1989; 4:506-511.
2. Greenfield S, Kaplan S, Ware J Jr. Expanding patient involvement in care: effects on patient outcomes. Ann Intern Med 1985; 102:520-528.
3. Korsch BM. What do patients and parents want to know? What do they need to know? Pediatrics 1984; 74:917-919.
4. Mahler HI, Kulik JA. Preferences for health care involvement, perceived control and surgical recovery: a prospective study. Soc Sci Med 1990; 31:743-751.
5. Ende J, Kazis L, Ash A et al. Measuring patients' desire for autonomy: decision making and information-seeking preferences among medical patients. J Gen Intern Med 1989; 4:23-30.
6. Waitzkin H. Doctor-patient communication: clinical implications of social scientific research. JAMA 1984; 252:2441-2446.
7. Llewellyn-Thomas HA, Thiel EC, Sem FWC et al. Presenting clinical trial information: a comparison of methods. Patient Educ Couns 1995; 25:97-107.
8. Gustafson DH, Bosworth K, Hawkins RP et al. CHESS: a computer-based support system for providing information, referrals, decision support and social support to people facing medical and other health-related crises. Proc Annu Symp Comput Appl Med Care 1992: 161-165.
9. Pingree S, Hawkins RP, Gustafson DH et al. Will HIV-positive people use an interactive computer system for information and support? A study of CHESS in two communities. Proc Annu Symp Comput Appl Med Care 1993:22-26.

10. Peterson C, Stunkard AJ. Personal control and health promotion. Soc Sci Med 1989; 28:819-828.
11. Cassileth B, Aupkis R, Sutton-Smith K et al. Information and participation preferences among cancer patients. Ann Intern Med 1980; 92:832-836.
12. Israel BA, Sherman SJ. Social support, control and the stress process. In: Glanz K, Lewis FM, Rimer B, eds. Health Behavior and Health Education. San Francisco, CA: Jossey-Bass, 1990.
13. Mullen PD, Laville EA, Biddle AK et al. Efficacy of psychoeducational interventions on pain, depression, and disability in people with arthritis: a meta-analysis. J Rheumatol 1987; 14(Suppl 15):33-39.
14. Maibach E, Flora J, Nass C. Changes in self-efficacy and health behavior in response to a minimal contact community health campaign. Health Communication 1991; 3:1-15.
15. Lorig K, Chastain RL, Ung E et al. Development and evaluation of a scale to measure perceived self-efficacy in people with arthritis. Arthritis Rheum 1989; 32:37-44.
16. Holman H, Lorig K. Patient education in the rheumatic diseases-pros and cons. Bull Rheum Dis 1987; 37:1-8.
17. Bandura A. Self-efficacy: towards a unifying theory of behavioral change. Psychol Rev 1977; 84:191-215.
18. O'Leary A, Shoor S, Lorig K et al. A cognitive-behavioral treatment for rheumatoid arthritis. Health Psychol 1988; 7:527-544.
19. Feste C, Anderson RM. Empowerment: from philosophy to practice. Patient Educ Couns 1995; 26:139-144.
20. Anderson RM, Funnell MM, Butler PM et al. Patient empowerment. Results of a randomized trial. Diabetes Care 1995; 18:943-949.
21. Allen JK, Becker DM, Swank RT. Factors related to functional status after coronary artery bypass surgery. Heart Lung 1990; 19:337-343.
22. Cunningham AJ, Lockwood GA, Cunningham JA. A relationship between perceived self-efficacy and quality of life in cancer patients. Patient Educ Couns 1991; 17:71-78.
23. O'Leary A. Self-efficacy and health. Behav Res Ther 1985; 23:437-451.
24. Gustafson DH, Hawkins RP, Boberg EW et al. The impact of computer support on HIV infected individuals. Final report to the Agency for Health Care Policy and Research 1994.
25. Jimison HB, Henrion M. Hierarchical preference models for patients with chronic disease. Med Decis Making 1992; 7:351.
26. Goldstein MK, Clarke AE, Michelson D et al. Developing and testing a multimedia presentation of a health-state description. Med Decis Making 1994; 14:336-344.
27. Nease RF Jr. Risk attitudes in gambles involving length of life: aspirations, variations, and ruminations. Med Decis Making 1994; 14:201-203.
28. Skinner CS, Strecher VJ, Hospers H. Physicians' recommendations for mammography: do tailored messages make a difference? Am J Public Health 1994; 84:43-49.

29. Thompson SC, Pitts JS, Schwankovsky L. Preferences for involvement in medical decision-making: situational and demographic influences. Patient Educ Couns 1993; 22:133-140.

30. Funnell MM, Donnelly MB, Anderson RM et al. Perceived effectiveness, cost, and availability of patient education methods and materials. Diabetes Educ 1992; 18:139-145.

31. Alterman AI, Baughman TG. Videotape versus computer interactive education in alcoholic and nonalcoholic controls. Alcoholism 1991; 15:39-44.

32. Gillispie MA, Ellis LBM. Computer-based patient education revisited. J Med Syst 1993; 17:119-125.

33. Consoli SM, Ben Said M, Jean J et al. Benefits of a computer-assisted education program for hypertensive patients compared with standard education tools. Patient Educ Couns 1995; 26:343-347.

34. Skinner CS, Siegfried JC, Kegler MC et al. The potential of computers in patient education. Patient Educ Couns 1993; 22:27-34.

35. Kasper JF, Mulley AF Jr., Wennberg JE. Developing shared decision making programs to improve the quality of health care. Qual Rev Bull 1992; 18:183-190.

36. Brown MS. Polish and glitz aside, net resources fall short on the content yardstick. Medicine on the Net 1996; 2:7-8.

37. Hubbard SM, Martin NB, Thurn AL. NCI's cancer information systems—bringing medical knowledge to clinicians. Oncology 1995; 9:302-309.

38. Ferguson CH. Computers and the coming of the U.S. keiretsu. Harv Bus Rev 1990; 68:55-70.

39. Kieschnick T, Adler L, Jimison HB. 1996 Health Informatics Directory. Baltimore, MD: Williams and Wilkins, 1995.

40. Jimison HB, Sher PP. Consumer health informatics: health information technology for consumers. J Am Soc Inf Sci 1995; 46:783-790.

41. Kreps GL. Communication and health education: systems and applications. In: Brand R, Donohew L, eds. Communication and Health: Systems and Applications. Hillsdale, NJ: Lawrence Erlbaum Associates, 1990.

42. Beisecker AE, Beisecker TD. Patient information-seeking behaviors when communicating with doctors. Med Care 1990; 28:19-28.

43. Kahn G. Computer-based patient education: a progress report. MD Comput 1993; 10:93-99.

44. Kahn G. Computer-generated patient handouts. MD Comput 1993; 10:157-164.

45. Bouhaddou O, Warner H. An interactive patient information and education system (Medical HouseCall) based on a physician expert system (Illiad). MedInfo 1995; 8 Pt 2:1181-1185.

46. Bouhaddou O, Lambert JG, Morgan GE. Illiad and Medical HouseCall: evaluating the impact of common sense knowledge on the diagnostic accuracy of a medical expert system. Proc Annu Symp Comput Appl Med Care 1995:742-746.

47. Peterson MC, Holbrook JH, Von Hales D et al. Contributions of the history, physical examination, and laboratory investigation in making medical diagnoses. West J Med 1992; 156:163-166.
48. Harris J. National Assessment of Consumer Health Information Demand and Delivery. in Summary Conference Report, Reference Point Foundation, Partnership for Networked Health Information for the Public, Rancho Mirage, CA. May 14-16, 1995. Washington, DC: Office of Disease Prevention and Health Promotion, DHHS, 1995, 3-5.
49. Davis TC, Crouch MA, Wills G et al. The gap between patient reading comprehension and the readability of patient education materials. J Fam Pract 1990; 31:533-538.
50. Doak CC, Doak LG, Root JH. Teaching Patients with Low Literacy Skills. Philadelphia: JB Lippincott, 1985.
51. Holt GA, Hallon JD, Hughes SE et al. OTC labels: can consumers read and understand them? Am Pharm 1990; 30:51-54.
52. Davis TC, Mayeaux EJ. Reading ability of parents compared with reading level of pediatric patient education materials. Pediatrics 1994; 93:460-468.
53. Petterson T. How readable are the hospital information leaflets available to elderly patients? Age Ageing 1994; 23:14-16.
54. Morgan PP. Illiteracy can have major impact on patients' understanding of health care information. Can Med Assoc J 1993; 148:1196-1197.
55. Feldman SR, Quinlivan A. Illiteracy and the readability of patient education materials. A look at Health Watch. N C Med J 1994; 55:290-292.
56. Jubelirer SJ, Linton JC. Reading versus comprehension: implications for patient education and consent in an outpatient oncology clinic. J Cancer Educ 1994; 9:26-29.
57. Reid JC, Klachko DM, Kardash CA et al. Why people don't learn from diabetes literature: influence of text and reader characteristics. Patient Educ Couns 1995; 25:31-38.
58. Berner ES, Webster GD, Shugerman AA et al. Performance of four computer-based diagnostic systems. N Engl J Med 1994; 330:1792-1796.
59. Sobel DS. Self-care in health: Information to empower people. In: Levy AH, Williams B. Proc Annu Conf—Am Assoc Med Syst Inf Conf 1987:12-125.

Part III

Future Development of Clinical Diagnostic Decision Support Systems

====== CHAPTER 7 ======

Design and Implementation Issues

Jerome H. Carter

The early 1970s were a time of great optimism for researchers in the field of medical artificial intelligence. The initial successes of systems such as MYCIN,[1] CASNET[2] and the Leeds abdominal pain system[3] made it reasonable to assume that it was only a matter of time until computers became a standard part of physicians' diagnostic armamentarium. As the other chapters in this book have shown, there have been a number of successful applications developed, many of which show promise for making a significant impact on patient care. However, after two decades of development of these programs no clinical diagnostic decision support system (CDDSS) is widely used by physicians. This chapter will examine some of the system design and implementation concerns that must be addressed if these systems are to realize their potential.

What accounts for this lack of use? The 30 year experience described by Engle[4] provides valuable insight into the problems encountered in the creation and deployment of diagnostic systems. He provides a list of factors divided into critical and noncritical, which he feels account for the difficulties in building a useful system and the rejection of diagnostic systems by clinicians. According to Engle, "Factors that play a role but are not critical include inadequate computers, and peripheral devices, difficulty some people have working with computers, systems not user-friendly, physicians' high regard for their own capabilities, and fear of computer competition, as well as the limited nature of the programs. In our estimation, the critical impediment to the development of decision programs useful in medicine lies in the impossibility of developing an adequate database and an effective set of decision rules." The findings of Berner et al.[5] help us understand some of the frustration noted by Engle. In their test of four general diagnostic systems, it was found that "...the proportion of correct diagnoses ranged from 0.52-0.71 and the mean proportion of relevant diagnoses ranged from 0.19-0.37..." This is hardly the type of performance which encourages use by a busy clinician. While this level of performance may be problematic for the broad-based systems like QMR,[6] Iliad[7] and DXplain,[8] programs with more limited domains such as Pathfinder[9] and the Leeds abdominal pain system[3] have been noted to perform very well. However, Shortliffe[10] properly notes that systems dedicated to a single problem tend to discourage wide usage because of their limited scope.

Another major design issue is the lack of integration into standard information systems;[10-12] thus tedious and time-consuming data entry is required. In contrast to the acceptance of diagnostic expert systems in the field of medicine, other disciplines have readily adopted them. DENDRAL,[13] which suggests the structure of organic molecules and R1[14] a system created by Digital Equipment Corporation which assists in the set up of computer systems have enjoyed broad support. The capability of DENDRAL, R1 and limited domain medical systems such as Pathfinder, demonstrates that decision support systems are feasible for routine usage in limited domains. Thus the question remains, what must be done in order to achieve success in broader problem areas? An excellent introduction to the matter is provided by Russell and Norvig[15] who point out that the field of medicine, unlike organic chemistry, lacks a general theoretical model. Also, medical diagnosis is fraught with uncertainty. Luger and Stubblefield[16] take the analysis further and identify five "deficiencies" of expert systems technology in general, which pose particular problems in judgment-related fields such as medicine. They are summarized below:

1. Lack of "deep"(causal) knowledge of the domain (i.e., systems do not understand physiology);
2. Lack of robustness and flexibility. Systems, when faced with a problem not contained in their knowledge bases cannot: solve the problem, recognize their inability to solve the problem, nor develop a strategy for doing so;

3. Inability to provide deep explanations;
4. Difficulties in verification;
5. Systems do not learn from experience.

The inability to reason with specialized data types (e.g., temporal, spatial), is another obvious shortcoming of many CDDSS. As discussed elsewhere in this book and in other literature, most systems have serious weaknesses in these areas. The issues mentioned thus far that need to be addressed in order for CDDSS to become more widely used may be divided into three broad categories: (1) technical design issues (reasoning methods, knowledge representation and acquisition); (2) human-computer interaction; and (3) systems integration. Each of these topics will be discussed in this chapter.

TECHNICAL DESIGN ISSUES

ADDING STRUCTURE TO MEDICAL KNOWLEDGE

In order to perform their desired tasks, CDDSS require access to knowledge about their domains. Facts, unadorned, relate little information about the world. Meaning requires an understanding of relationships. Seeing the number 17,000 as an isolated value carries no message. However, once it is related to a modifier, "white blood cell count," it has clinical meaning. The goal of knowledge representation is to provide intelligent systems with information about a specific domain in a form that can be processed efficiently. The representational scheme along with domain facts together constitute a knowledge base. Over the last 20 years, researchers have created a number of representational schemes ranging from simple collections of logic predicates to elaborate network structures. The expressive power of the representational scheme chosen for an intelligent system has direct bearing on the types of problems the system may be expected to solve, as well as how it goes about solving them. For example, a system for detecting and warning about potential drug interactions needs a way of representing drug classes, alternate names for medications, and the difference between drugs that are topical and those that are introduced into the body. If we were to decide later that predicting the ultimate effect of a drug on a clinical state is the desired output, temporal and physiologic information must be somehow represented in our knowledge base. Logic-based reasoning would work well for the first system; the second would require a causal mechanism.

KNOWLEDGE REPRESENTATION FORMATS

Most knowledge representation schemes fall into one of four categories: logic, procedural, graph/network, or structured. Although not considered a classic architecture for knowledge bases, database management systems will undoubtedly play a significant role in this arena as more clinical information systems use this format for data storage. The following discussion reviews some of the concepts discussed in chapter 2 and illustrates additional knowledge representation schemes.

Logic-Based Knowledge Representation

Propositional logic was the first representational format widely used for artificial intelligence research. As previously discussed in chapter 2, propositions are statements about the world that are either true or false. These statements may be connected together to form sentences. Each statement may then be represented by a letter such as "P". To illustrate, consider the two propositions "the MCV is decreased in iron deficiency anemia" and "the MCV is increased in pernicious anemia". The first statement is represented as "P" and the second as "Q". Propositional logic provides rules for manipulating statements: "P and Q," "P or Q," "P and not (Q)," are legal sentences.

The statements which we have asserted concerning the relationship between the MCV and anemia are useful; however, they must be used as whole statements, i.e., we cannot take pernicious anemia from Q and use it to form new assertions. First-order logic (first-order predicate calculus) does offer this option. Predicate calculus provides a means of representing logic statements in a way that permits components of the assertion to be used as variables. We are no longer stuck with just "P and Q". Using predicate calculus, the anemia propositions may be rewritten as:

MCV (increased, pernicious anemia)
MCV (decreased, iron deficiency).

Now MCV appears as a "predicate" which provides information concerning the relationship of the "objects" it acts on (increased and pernicious anemia in the first example). In this form questions can be asked of the type MCV (x, iron deficiency), which may read as "what is the value of the MCV in iron deficiency anemia"? This new flexibility, the ability to add predicates to a knowledge base and then to use those predicates to answer questions, provided a significant boost to the use of logic as a basis for expert system design. The programming language PROLOG (PROgramming in LOGic), which has been used to create a number of expert systems, was designed specifically to allow researchers to experiment with issues in the use of first-order predicate calculus as a knowledge representation format.

Procedural Knowledge Representations

Logic-based representations are declarative in nature, in that they consist of true or false statements and all questions are resolved through standard logic inferencing mechanisms. In a logic based system the diagnosis of anemia associated with "increased" MCV would be made by looking through all the "MCV" logic predicates and finding those that have "increased" as an object. All matching predicates would then be returned (in this case there is only one such predicate, pernicious anemia). Procedural formats, on the other hand, provide more explicit information about how the knowledge base is to be used to answer a question, it is not simply a "look up" of known facts. A procedural recasting of the anemia facts would yield:

IF MCV is increased
THEN conclude pernicious anemia

IF MCV is decreased
THEN conclude iron deficiency anemia

Notice that procedural systems offer a "process" of sorts to aid in making the diagnosis (i.e., they tell how to use the facts to draw a conclusion). These process statements are provided in the form of rules. Rule-based systems are prototypical procedural representations and have been the dominant format for medical expert systems since the days of MYCIN.[1]

Networks

Networks are specialized structures consisting of nodes (representing facts, events, objects, processes, etc.) and arcs which link the nodes. As described in chapter 2, Bayesian belief networks have proven to be very capable representation schemes for probabilistic reasoning systems, overcoming earlier objections to simple Bayesian expert systems. The flexibility of the network paradigm has greatly increased its popularity over the past fifteen years. For instance, nodes in a network might consist of frames as advocated by Minsky, or other structures. Even more significant is the capacity of networks to capture causal, temporal and other hard-to-model knowledge quite readily.

Decision trees[17] and artificial neural networks[18] are other types of network representation schemes which have recently come into favor with CDDSS designers. They will be discussed in more detail later.

DATA REPRESENTATION

Structural representations emphasize the "packaging" of knowledge into well defined pieces with higher levels of organization. The first widely adopted structural format was the "frame" metaphor created by Minsky.[19] Frames are complex data structures which contain information about the concept being described along with procedural information detailing how the frame may change over time. For example, the concept "grocery shopping" may be represented as:

Concept: Grocery Shopping
Location: Supermarket
Actions: Item selection (procedure)
Paying (procedure)

Database management systems (DBMS) offer another structured format for knowledge representation. There are two types of databases which are found frequently in clinical settings—relational and object oriented. Relational databases are based on a record structure in which each record has a number of fields. A primary field is designated and all remaining fields in the record are related directly to this primary field. A disease record might have the following fields:

Disease Name, Organ System, Diagnostic Test, Gender Affected.
Disease (Disease Name, Organ System, Diagnostic Test, Gender Affected)

Records are then collected together into tables. Each row in the table represents a unique record and each column a feature of the record as illustrated below in Table 7.1.

Additional columns could be used to improve the richness of the disease description. Each column in a relational record holds a specific type of data (e.g., number, text, boolean). However, a column

Table 7.1. Example of a disease record table

Disease Name	Organ System	Dx Tests	Gender
Pneumonia	Respiratory	X-Ray	Both
Hypothyroidism	Endocrine	TSH	Both

cannot hold more complex data structures, for example, another record, or a list of numbers. Object-oriented database management systems (OODBMS) permit greater expressiveness by permitting the storage of data types which cannot be handled by relational, table-based systems.[20]

An anemia object might be defined as follows:

System:	hematological
Anemia Type:	microcytic, hypochromic
Disease:	iron deficiency anemia
Tests:	list (serum iron, TIBC, ferritin)
Rx:	ferrous sulfate, ferrous gluconate
Picture:	(binary) peripheral smear

This anemia object contains a "list" (a collection of facts or objects) and a picture as fields in a record (this feature is rarely seen in relational systems). More importantly, objects can "inherit" traits thereby permitting new objects to be defined in terms of those which currently exist. This allows for the creation of new data types, a feature which is not found in purely relational systems. OODBMS have already begun to be used by researchers designing decision support systems and hold great promise for use in clinical information systems.[21]

Structured query language (SQL) may be used to "ask" questions of a database; however, SQL does not support the creation of inferences, i.e., the ability to draw inferences from the data. A major drawback to using a database as a knowledge base is the lack of a specific knowledge processing mechanism for these systems. However, the ability to use higher level computer languages with database files lessens the significance of this deficiency. Still, adding inferencing capabilities is not a trivial task.

SPECIAL DATA TYPES

Providing support for medical diagnostic decisions presents unique problems to system designers because of the size of the problem domain. Adding to the situation is the need to provide knowledge about dynamic states. This requires not only facts about the objects themselves (diseases, tests, drugs, etc.) but also, information concerning how these things might change over time. Predicting metastasis requires anatomical knowledge about circulation patterns and "next to" and "behind" facts. Understanding the possible effect of a medication requires knowledge of physiology (elimination times, routes, distribution, etc.). The need for causal, temporal and spatial knowledge is a major challenge for system designers. There remains no widely accepted format for representing the passage of time, three-dimensional anatomical relationships, nor physiological information. Programs such as ABEL, CASNET and CHF advisor[2,22,23] have made some progress with causal knowledge representation; however, no "portable," generalized representation is extant.

The effective handling of temporal knowledge has been an important AI research area from the beginning. Allen[24] was the first to offer a formalism for handling temporal data. He presented a format based on time points and intervals. However, the method proposed by Allen is felt to be computationally intractable when used to explain all possible relations between a set of actions and processes.[25] Appropriate handling of temporal information requires not only a means of representing instants and intervals, but also a formal means of representing the temporal concepts commonly used by humans. The passage of time, of which humans have an innate understanding, is not so easily represented in digital format. Basic temporal concepts such as distinguishing between future and past events, time dependency (i.e., did event X occur 3 minutes, 3 days or 3 years before event Y), and concurrency (while X is occurring Y usually happens) are essential if CDDSS are to reason about prognosis, outcomes, toxicities, etc. Medical artificial intelligence (AI) researchers have created a variety of temporal representation and reasoning methods to deal these issues. Shahar and Musen[25] offer a closed-interval, discrete model based upon intervals and time points. Events are represented as intervals. Intervals may have attached parameter value which can be numerical (primitive) or qualitative (abstract). There are three types of abstracted intervals: state, gradient and rate. The RESUME system which embodies this model also includes a temporal inference mechanism and truth maintenance system which ensures that any changes to primitive data is reflected throughout the system. TOPAZ, a system developed by Kahn et al.,[26] which analyzes the temporal sequences of white blood cell counts and chemotherapy drug dosing, also makes use of intervals to represent temporal events in association with causal physiologic data. Kohane[27] provides a third example of encoding temporal information. His experience with adding temporal information to a knowledge base points out a final issue with using temporal data. He states, "The addition of temporal information to medical knowledge bases requires significant effort. In my experience of developing modestly sized knowledge bases...the task of adding temporal constraints to every event equaled that of building the rest of the knowledge base."

All of the temporal models discussed thus far are explicit representations, whereas most diagnostic systems encode temporal data implicitly. Aliferis et al.[28] address the issue of the need for explicit temporal models and inferencing mechanisms. They note that systems such as QMR, Iliad and MYCIN manage to function quite well within their domains without having specific mechanisms for dealing with temporal data. They go on to argue that no formal theoretical or empirical argument has been made concerning the relative value of using explicit vs. implicit temporal models. It is very possible that explicit temporal modeling is more important for some types of decision support activities (prognosis, outcomes research) than for others (diagnosis) based upon the character of the knowledge bases. Perhaps systems that rely upon frequently changing clinical data require explicit mechanisms for handling time dependent data, whereas those with more static knowledge bases and which rely on human input can perform quite well with implicit characterizations. Either way, much needs to be done in this area.

Default Knowledge

There are a number of important problems in knowledge representation and knowledge base design that are independent of format—inconsistency, degree of expressiveness, and incompleteness are ready examples. The most interesting, and without doubt one of the most difficult to solve, is that of default or commonsense knowledge. There are facts about humans which clinicians, when discussing patient problems, consider too basic to even mention—females become pregnant, men get prostate cancer. Default reasoning may be viewed as a means of dealing with incompleteness.[29] Consider the statement, "The patient in room 574 is 6 months pregnant." Automatically it can be determined (by a human) that this patient: (1) needs yearly Papanicolaou smears; (2) should not receive certain medications; and (3) will have an abrupt decrease in weight in 3 months or so. If our knowledge base had contained the fact 'males do not become pregnant' and did not have a 'females become pregnant' fact, a default reasoning system might gracefully default to 'the patient in room 574 is female' and proceed with its analysis. This approach to incompleteness is not without problems. Ponder the effect of a drug dosing system that gives a medication because no statement of patient allergy is found in its knowledge base. How should default information be encoded and used? Proposed solutions to this problem will be discussed later in this chapter.

REASONING

Due to the fact that early systems were designed by researchers interested in "artificial intelligence," much of the work on diagnostic expert systems was aimed at getting these systems to mimic the decision-making processes of human experts. Interestingly, programs such as MYCIN, Pathfinder and the Leeds system, while quite capable, do not "reason" in the same manner as humans. They have no innate understanding of human anatomy or physiology, are unable to handle temporal concepts, and have no ability to learn or deduce new facts. Yet, within their narrow domain, it has been demonstrated that they can perform comparably to human experts. However, once the domain of expected expertise is broadened, performance significantly worsens. The failure of techniques used in the design of limited domain systems to "scale up" to more general systems is a major driving force behind current research in medical artificial intelligence and by extension, CDDSS. The ability to reason from "first principles" and to understand the effects of time on disease processes, are considered essential to building robust systems which have more human-like capabilities. Over the last 20 years a significant amount of work has been done in the area of causal modeling (i.e., addition of anatomical and physiological data to knowledge bases).[2,22,23] Temporal reasoning and representation have also received a good deal of attention.[25-27] Aside from adding human-like abilities, issues such as the computational burden of large numbers of calculations in networks, handling conflicting rules in knowledge bases, gracefully handling uncertainty and ignorance, and methodologies for acquiring new knowledge, are sufficiently formidable so as to attract the attention of researchers. We will begin the exploration of these issues with the problem of reasoning.

RULE-BASED AND EARLY BAYESIAN SYSTEMS

In order to understand the research issues related to reasoning, it is necessary to trace the development of inference mechanisms in CDDSS. The most basic inference mechanism utilized in medical diagnostic systems is propositional logic. In systems of this type knowledge is stored in the form of facts. An example of a knowledge base consisting of only two facts might be: "CPK-MB is increased in myocardial infarction (MI)" and "chest pain is present in MI". All facts concerning the findings associated with myocardial infarctions would, coupled with a mechanism for testing their validity, allow one to draw a conclusion about the presence of an MI in a patient. For example, if we state as a premise that "patient x has chest pain and an increased serum CPK-MB," it would be reasonable to conclude that the patient had an MI. This may be written in the form:

IF patient x has
chest pain and
CPK-MB is increased
THEN the problem is MI

Notice that our small knowledge base does not contain any facts about other possible causes of chest pain; therefore, the system could not conclude that the patient has esophageal reflux. According to Russell and Norvig,[15] logic systems have three properties which are particularly useful. We will make use of only one of them for this discussion—'locality'. If there is a statement of the form "if a then b" and "a" is known to be true, then we can conclude that "b" is true regardless of whatever else is known to be true. Locality is very useful in logic systems where all facts are either completely true or completely false (for this discussion being true is equivalent to "is only caused by" and false "is never caused by"). However, in the field of medicine, there are very few findings which can be so neatly categorized. Consider what happens when we add the fact "chest pain is present in esophageal reflux." The presence of chest pain no longer absolutely implies MI. Locality no longer holds. Rule-based systems such as MYCIN inherit the properties of logic systems and the possibility of inconsistency in the knowledge base. The fundamental issue becomes one of handling uncertainty gracefully. Finally, Russell and Norvig offer three reasons why most systems based on propositional logic are unworkable for medical diagnosis. These reasons are related to the unavoidable presence of uncertainty; Russell and Norvig describe them as laziness, theoretical ignorance, and practical ignorance. Laziness, in this instance, describes the reluctance of system designers to do the work necessary to "list a complete set of antecedents or consequents needed to ensure an exceptionless rule and it is too hard to use the enormous rules that result." Theoretical ignorance is simply an acknowledgment that there is no theory of medicine to guide modeling of the domain. Last, practical ignorance is a statement of the fact that, for any particular patient, even if we knew all the applicable rules, we would rarely have access to all the required information (tests, genetic history, etc.).

MYCIN pioneered the use of 'certainty factors'—numerical estimates of the confidence in a particular fact. They are based upon the opinions of domain experts and are not derived from epidemiological data. Certainty factors can take on values from -1 (indicating certainty that a condition is not true) to 1 that it is true. Zero indicates that little is known about a particular fact. This is an important feature which differentiates them from true probability estimates which must be between 0 and 1. For example, we could add certainty factors to our MI knowledge base:

> IF chest pain is present
> THEN conclude MI .65

Certainty factors were an attempt to deal with uncertainty. However, as will be illustrated, their use in a rule-based, logic derived system may lead to erroneous conclusions.

Consider the effect of adding the rule:

> IF chest pain is present
> THEN conclude esophageal reflux .40

In a system where locality is expected, if rule 1 fires, then "conclude MI .65" will become the active hypothesis. Yet it is possible that rule 2 may also be valid. In order to arrive at the correct diagnosis some mechanism must be in place to adjudicate between the two rules or the knowledge base designers must ensure that the two rules will never conflict. In a domain such as medicine, where thousands of rules may be needed, it is easy to see how conflicts might creep into the knowledge base and undermine the accuracy of the system. An excellent discussion of the failings of rule-based systems using certainty factors may be found in Heckerman et al.[9]

Unlike MYCIN, the Leeds abdominal pain system was based on simple Bayesian computation. However, early Bayesian systems had their own problems. The most significant was the number of probability estimates required to make the system workable. In addition, each new piece of evidence required recalculation of all pertinent probability estimates resulting in a burdensome number of computations. A final requirement of early Bayesian systems was "conditional independence" (an assumption that all relationships between evidence and hypothesis are independent). The inability to assure conditional independence caused Bayesian reasoning systems to lose favor with expert system developers. Thus, even though MYCIN and the Leeds system proved to be capable of performing well within their problem domains, their reasoning mechanisms were considered to be inadequate for larger problems.

CAUSAL REASONING

Causal reasoning, simply defined, is the use of deep domain knowledge (i.e., pathophysiology, anatomy, etc.) to assist in the decision making process. The fact that clinicians, when faced with a difficult problem, also resort to this form of reasoning served to enhance its attractiveness as a model for inferencing in CDDSS. Patil[30] argues very cogently on behalf of causal reasoning as a guiding principle in CDDSS. He offers a few of the potential benefits—describing the evolution of diseases over time, reasoning about interactions among diseases, and the ability to understand specific mechanisms.

CASNET[2] was the first medical expert system based upon causal precepts. Designed to assist in the diagnosis of glaucoma, CASNET's knowledge is represented in the system as a network of pathophysiologic states. A particularly interesting feature of CASNET is the hierarchical organization of its knowledge base. At the lowest level are patient signs, symptoms and tests. The middle layer consists of pathophysiologic states such as corneal edema and elevated intraocular pressure. The highest knowledge level is composed of disease categories—open angle glaucoma, secondary glaucoma, etc. Connections between the layers represent direct causal relationships, allowing diseases at the highest level to be viewed as aggregations of patient findings and pathophysiologic states. Reasoning is carried out by navigating a path from findings to disease, testing pathway nodes by calculating a likelihood value for each then following the highest likelihood pathway.

The CHF Advisor[22] and ABEL[23] represent alternate approaches to causal reasoning. The CHF Advisor, which assists with the diagnosis and management of heart failure, is based upon a qualitative physiologic model of the cardiovascular system. A truth-maintenance system (TMS) enforces relationships between parameters. The TMS also allows the program to test the effects of changes in a particular variable on the entire model. This permits one to experiment with the effects of altering the value of various parameters.

ABEL has acid-base and electrolyte disorders as its domain. ABEL's knowledge base, like CASNET, models its domain at three levels of detail. Its highest level represents clinical states (i.e., hypokalemia, acidosis) while the lowest level is a physiologic representation of electrolyte stores and movement between various fluid compartments. As noted by Patil,[30] "The critical feature of ABEL is its ability to determine and represent situations where a hypothesis is capable of explaining part but not all of an observed finding." Limited causal modeling has been used in systems such as Caduceus.[31] Causal links are implemented in the knowledge base in the form of "may be caused by" relationships, serving to constrain the number of nodes evaluated during the diagnostic process. The causal links in Caduceus are much more primitive than those in ABEL, CASNET and CHF Advisor in that they do not represent deep knowledge of the domain. The use of a more superficial form of causal links has been exploited in a newer type of diagnostic system, belief networks, which will be discussed in a later section.

Causal reasoning, while effective, does have significant limitations as an inference mechanism. The lack of knowledge concerning the actual mechanism for a number of diseases remains a major impediment to the creation of causal systems—i.e., the pathophysiology of rheumatologic disorders is much less well defined than those in cardiology. Thus, general domain systems such as QMR cannot be completely built using this reasoning model. However, this does not preclude the inclusion of causal knowledge in these systems. In fact a good deal of causal knowledge is encoded implicitly in QMR's knowledge base.

Another design issue for causal systems is level of detail. ABEL has three levels of detail represented in its knowledge base. How many should be included to be considered complete? Is a complete representation possible or even desirable? Perhaps the ultimate design issue is that of "understanding." CASNET and ABEL are designed as networks of causally linked nodes. And although they can use deep knowledge of their domains, they do not understand what they are manipulating (the "holy grail" of AI research from the beginning).

A final matter is that of temporal representation in causal networks. One of the most basic aspects of any disease is the temporal relationship among findings. If one knew that a mass has been present on a chest radiograph for 15 years, it would automatically be considered benign. What is the best way to represent the implausibility of this being malignant in a knowledge base? All of these questions add complexity to the design process.

PROBABILISTIC REASONING

Bayesian reasoning systems fell out of favor in the mid 1970's due to the need to develop and maintain huge probability tables (joint probability distributions) in order to perform the required calculations. Aside from the need to maintain probability distribution data, a separate and equally daunting problem was that of assuring conditional independence of findings. In many cases, especially for any sufficiently large domain, this was difficult to achieve. A solution to both problems was advanced by the findings of a number of researchers in the form of belief networks.[9,32,33]

A belief network is a directed acyclic graph (the arrows point in one direction and there are no circular paths) consisting of nodes which contain conditional probability data. Nodes may be thought of as "parent" and "child" with parent nodes connected to child nodes by one-way arrows. Conditional probability tables at each node reflect the effect of all the parent nodes on the child node. As might be expected, even this format is computationally intensive for all but small networks. If you will recall, one of the problems of early Bayesian systems was conditional independence. This criticism is addressed by network designers via the use of causal relationships when creating networks and by use of a catch-all probability estimate in the form of a "noise parameter." If we say the probability of MI is .7 given finding X and .2 given finding Y, then .3 represents the noise for X and .8 for Y. Conditional independence values are not exact, but the use of noisiness permits usable systems to be built.[34] Heckerman et al. achieved an acceptable solution by building a limited number of conditional dependencies into their Pathfinder Network.[9] Judea Pearl has produced an excellent text on this subject for those who wish to develop a fuller understanding of this area.[35]

Decision-Theoretic Reasoning

A relatively recent innovation in medical expert systems design is the use of decision theory in the reasoning process.[36,37] Decision theory is based upon the concept of utility—the value to the decision maker of a particular outcome. In the case of a patient with chest pain where either esophageal reflux or MI might be the cause, a pure probabilistic system would offer as its conclusion the diagnosis with the highest probability (for the sake of argument assume that this is reflux). In a decision-theoretic system, the cost to the patient of suggesting reflux when the correct diagnosis is MI would be calculated before offering a final conclusion. Thus utility serves to "remind" the system of the "cost" of an incorrect diagnosis or suggested action. A significant problem with decision-theoretic systems is that of determining how the utilities included in a system will be determined— never a simple undertaking. Nevertheless, this is a promising development in the design of decision support systems.

"Possibilistic" Reasoning

The discussion of reasoning thus far has focused on the handling of uncertainty. Uncertainty is an expression of the inability to know all the factors involved in a particular decision and their ultimate effect upon the outcome. Lofti Zadeh pointed out another decision making dilemma—imprecision in the expression of a finding or factor.[38,39] The statement, 'cervical cancer is a disease of younger women' is an example of fuzziness. At what age does a woman stop being young? Zadeh proposed that unlike traditional set theory in which an element was in only one set, membership may be possible to some extent in a number of sets. Thus a 35-year-old woman would have partial membership in the old set (say 0.3) as well as in the young set (0.7). Fuzzy logic provides a formalism for computing the truthfulness of fuzzy propositions. Maiers has written a good review of fuzzy logic in medical expert systems.[40]

Accounting for Ignorance

Dempster and Shafer[41] proposed a theory of evidence as a means of dealing with ignorance, as opposed to uncertainty. Their proposal arose out of the difficulty of assigning prior probability values. In most situations, these values are estimates and therefore subject to error. The Dempster-Shafer theory proposes that probability estimates be qualified by using a "belief function" which computes one's belief in a particular proposition. Belief functions add to the computational complexity of a system and due to their weaker theoretical grounding (as compared to Bayesian and fuzzy systems) have received less support among CDDSS designers.

Commonsense Reasoning

Commonsense reasoning, at its most basic level, is about making assumptions. This is an indispensable capability that we use constantly. Commonsense (default) reasoning allows objects to be grouped into recognizable classes which can be mentally manipulated based on common traits. For example, birds fly, cars use gasoline, and planes land only at airports are statements about classes of objects that are well defined. If one is then told that a car would not run, an automatic question would be whether it is out of gas. Now consider what happens when decisions have been made using the facts mentioned previously, and it is discovered that electric cars and emus exist. What should be done? Should all prior decisions be revised? How should these new facts be added to the knowledge base? New facts concerning objects currently represented in the knowledge base must be reconciled with those already present. How should precedence be determined? Also, how should conclusions added to the knowledge base under the influence of old rules be updated or retracted? Default logic as suggested by Reiter[29] and the nonmonotonic logic of McDermott[42] are offered as reasoning mechanisms to deal with these problems. However, no system is available which adequately addresses all issues. In addition, no working CDDSS have been designed using default reasoning mechanisms.

CASED-BASED REASONING

Cased-based systems offer an approach to learning and reasoning that is very different from those discussed previously. A case, as defined by Kolodner,[43] is "a contextualized piece of knowledge representing an experience that teaches a lesson fundamental to achieving the goals of the reasoner." Case-based knowledge bases have two distinct parts: the case itself and an index that aids efficient context-based retrieval. Case-based systems acquire knowledge by solving problems. Cases are stored knowledge that reflect past experience in solving problems. Each case has three components—problem/situation description, solution, and outcome. The problem-situation-description describes the past situation or problem that was solved. It also includes the goals of the reasoner as the problem was being solved, and information about the problem environment. The solution component contains information regarding how the problem was solved. The result of applying the solution, whether the attempt succeeded or failed, and why, are stored in the outcome component. Access to cases is controlled by an index. The key to solving problems in case-based systems is matching the current problem to past experience. Compared to more traditional approaches, advocates of case-based systems believe they have the following advantages: (1) they are better at solving problems with open-ended, poorly defined concepts; (2) they arrive at solutions faster; (3) they are better at solving problems where no good algorithm is available; and (4) cases may serve as explanations.

Case-based reasoning is not without problems, however. In a large knowledge base retrieval efficiency is an important determinant of performance. Therefore, indexing is a key research area. Issues such as whether to use high level or low level features when building indexes, how to design a general framework for index content, and the design of case retrieval algorithms remain a source of vexation for those designing case-based systems. Despite its problems, case-based reasoning has been used successfully in CDDSS[44,45] and offers an interesting metaphor for building flexible knowledge-based systems.

Neural Networks

Neural networks rely upon pattern recognition to arrive at conclusions. They are more interesting as a learning system than a reasoning mechanism and will be discussed below.

KNOWLEDGE ACQUISITION

Knowledge Engineering

Knowledge engineering is the process of building a knowledge base. A knowledge engineer is a professional with an understanding of issues in knowledge representation, tool selection, artificial intelligence (AI) languages and software design. A knowledge engineer works with a "domain expert" to obtain the necessary data to build a knowledge base (knowledge acquisition). This has been the traditional model for building expert systems. Knowledge engineering can be a very tedious process. For example, QMR's knowledge base has been under development since the 1970s and is not yet complete. The time required to build a knowledge base for any decent-sized domain is often considerable and greatly inhibits the production and deployment of knowledge based systems. Much of the difficulty in building expert systems in any domain is due to the lack of a well-defined process for the activity. Even with the availability of specialized shells, languages, and other tools, the knowledge extraction process is still haphazard. Domain experts can be very poor at describing what they do or how they approach a problem. The knowledge engineer often has to learn the domain in order to identify major unifying concepts. Next, the actual problem to be solved must be agreed upon, and finally, knowledge representation formats and a reasoning mechanism must be chosen. Errors made at any step can result in significant delays and frustrations. Once completed, maintenance becomes a serious problem which can worsen by turnover on the development team. The "knowledge acquisition bottleneck" has no real solution using traditional methods. Also, standard knowledge engineering practices do not take advantage of the gigabytes of data stored in information systems currently in use. As a result of these obstacles and recent discoveries, machine learning has become a hot topic in knowledge based systems design. Machine learning has been an area of intense research since the early days of artificial intelligence and a tremendous body of work on this topic has been produced. For our discussion, we will examine only those which have had an impact in the medical domain.

Types of Learning

Machine learning takes place in two types of environments: supervised and unsupervised. In supervised systems, a "trainer" provides examples to a system and provides information on how to determine the correct outputs. Unsupervised systems are also provided with training examples but are expected to classify the example without outside help. Only supervised learning systems will be discussed here.

Decision Trees

Decision trees operate as classifiers by accepting input and converting it into a pattern of binary response nodes. Starting at the highest level node, each node along a path is tested and a branch taken depending upon the value of the response. Due to their structure, decision trees are capable of representing only a single subject. A decision tree for diagnosing the cause of anemia might appear as pictured in Figure 7.1.

Decision trees are excellent tools for classification problems and have received a good deal of attention lately via the field of data mining (looking for patterns in large databases). The work by Quinlan[46] with the ID3 (Induction for Decision Trees) algorithm gave the field a tremendous boost. ID3 builds a decision tree by first ranking all features in a data set in terms of how well they separate out subsets of the group. The most effective feature is then used to form the root of the tree. In the anemia example, the "MCV" is the best feature for initial classification. The beauty of algorithms such as ID3 is that they can be used with very large data sets and have excellent performance. For example, a database containing all test results from a hematology lab could be used to train an ID3 based system to diagnose anemia. A newer, more powerful form of ID3, C4.5 has even better classification capability.

Even very powerful decision trees have significant limitations. They are obviously not suited to building complex causal representations. Also, they are limited to addressing one subject per tree and

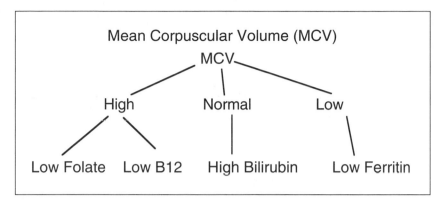

Fig. 7.1. Decision tree for diagnosis of anemia

they do not make any use of domain knowledge. However, the increasing use of databases in medicine assures that they will be valuable knowledge discovery tools.

Artificial Neural Networks

Artificial neural networks were briefly introduced in chapter 2. They are included here because of the learning capabilities they possess. Neural networks are based on concepts borrowed from neurobiology and in a very general way mimic the functioning of the brain. A common neural network architecture used for many decision support systems consists of multiple layers of similar elements. Each unit is called a neuron and is capable of receiving input (stimulation). When the total amount of stimulation received exceeds some predetermined threshold, the neuron "fires". A network consisting of layers of fully connected neurons is pictured below in Figure 7.2.

Each connection between units carries a value, referred to as a weight, which determines the amount of influence each neuron has on the other. Neural networks learn by being presented with data sets which contain the features of the problem to be solved. The trainer presents data (training set) to the network along with an example of the correct output. The most popular network training algorithm, back-propagation, trains the network by comparing the desired output provided by the trainer with that which the network generates. If there is a difference, the network determines the difference (a real number) and propagates that value from the output layer back to the

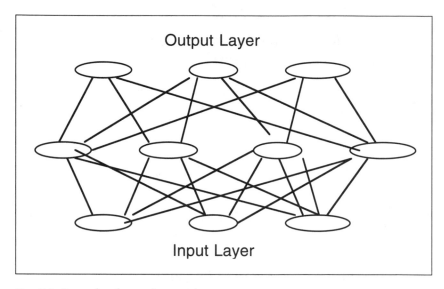

Fig. 7.2. Example of neural network

middle layer and then to the input level. Once all network outputs agree with those provided by the trainer, those network weights become fixed and the network is considered trained. Neural networks have been widely used for medical applications.[18,47-49] They are noted for their ability to learn patterns in data which is noisy (i.e., with missing or irregular elements). Analysis of their behavior indicates they function by doing a form of nonlinear regression. They are also excellent in situations where the trainer is unsure of the actual relationships which exist in the training set.

There are, however, a number of valid criticisms of neural network technology. The most important for AI researchers is that neural networks are, in essence, a "black box". Connection weights, which store the knowledge in neural networks, are determined internally during training and cannot be evaluated by humans. For example, in a neural net designed to diagnose anemia, there would be no particular "MCV" node. And no particular connection would code for the relationship between low MCV and low iron. Thus, even when a net performs perfectly it is not possible for the trainer to understand how the network arrives at its conclusions by examining the nodes and connections. The issue of network size is another problematic area.

Deciding on the size of a network (number of neurons and number of layers) is still very much an art form with no reliable algorithms to aid the process. A final criticism is that of training time. There is no process for assuring that a network can be trained in a given period of time, which can result in a good deal of frustration when attempting to utilize this technology.

Genetic Algorithms

Genetic algorithms (GAs) represent a significant departure from classic expert systems design. They do not make use of knowledge bases or reasoning mechanisms in the traditional sense. GAs use the principles of natural selection and genetics to generate "answers". Genetic algorithms are used for optimization problems. For example, given a multi-step treatment algorithm, what is the best combination of interventions which maximizes health status and minimizes costs? The solution is expressed in the form of a "chromosome" in which each possible step in the pathway is coded as a "gene". Solutions are generated by rearranging the genes (reproduction, crossover, mutation) on a chromosome and then testing the chromosome using a "fitness" algorithm. Much as the lack of robust learning algorithms limited the usefulness of early artificial neural networks, the difficulty of creating an effective fitness algorithm limits the application of genetic algorithms. Goldberg[30] provides an excellent tutorial on this subject.

HUMAN-COMPUTER INTERACTION

User Level Issues

It is now time to discuss the issues raised by Engle[4] and others concerning the lack of widespread use of decision support technology in clinical medicine. Heathfield and Wyatt,[12] provide an analysis of what they consider to be the psychological and organizational barriers that explain this situation. Their opinion is that most systems have not been designed to address the problems that clinicians actually face. They point out that several systems are designed to restrict the number of active diagnostic hypotheses (which doctors do quite well), while few are designed to help with differential diagnosis and treatment advice. The latter type have been much better received than the former. Identifying a well-defined problem to solve should be, but sometimes has not been, an important consideration for systems' designers.

CDDSS also must take clinicians' work habits into account. Systems must be available at the point of care and must be easy to use if they are to be considered clinical tools. The criticism offered by Clayton and Hripcsak[11] extends this analysis by noting that stand-alone systems which require significant data entry will not be used on any regular basis. Finally, the single-problem focus of many systems means that they will be needed only on rare occasions at which time it may not be worth the trouble to locate and use them. This could even be true of general systems covering multiple domains which, as Miller and Geissbuhler note in chapter 1, might only be justified in a small percentage of patients.

Problem Knowledge Couplers (PKCs), as advanced by Weed,[51] represent a rather unique approach to the use of diagnostic/therapeutic decision support. PKCs are intended to be used at the point-of-care and on a regular basis, not just for cases which are perceived to be diagnostically difficult. In fact, they are designed so that even nonmedical personnel can enter the patient's data, although the physician must still interpret the output. PKCs consist of an extensive knowledge base of diagnoses, findings and management options. Each individual coupler addresses a single presenting problem. The couplers permit controlled input of findings and guide the clinician in the process of diagnosis and management. PKC knowledge bases contain weighted findings (set by the coupler builder) which determine the display order of diagnostic and therapeutic suggestions.

PKCs are interesting from the standpoint of user interaction because they are meant to be an integral part of each clinical encounter. However, it is difficult to predict how widespread their use will become, since they represent a significant intrusion into the clinical practice environment and it is not clear that they will be useful for a large number of patients. For example, consider having a coupler for headache diagnosis and management. For most patients, an experienced clinician can easily differentiate between types of headaches based on clinical presentation. Using a coupler would be expected (as with other broad-domain systems) to be helpful for only a small number of cases. Thus the return for time invested, if used for every headache patient, would be very low.

Heathfield and Wyatt,[12] have identified several other problems systems' designers need to avoid. The first is a preoccupation with computer artifacts. In other words, when beginning a project there may be a tendency to focus more on what language to use, hardware configurations, and development environments than on the problems of potential users. Healthfield and Wyatt argue that this preoccupation can hamper the quest for the best problem-solving process and techniques for solving the particular problem.

Next they feel that system designers may fail to use appropriate models for solving problems and may fail to communicate clearly the design issues with potential users. This problem can be readily understood by any nontechnical person who has acted as a consultant for the development of a computer system, only to find that early on in the process the developers have lost all conception of what the ultimate product will be or how it will perform.

The final problem mentioned by Heathfield and Wyatt is that designers sometimes focus on system development and ignore organizational issues. Organizational attitudes and support play a critical role in the development and implementation of any technology. The multidisciplinary nature of CDDSS development makes this process even more vulnerable to problems of changing personnel, funding, administrative buy-in, and shifting organizational goals. Successful deployment of CDDSS technology requires that all these matters be addressed via a specific organizational policy for the creation and utilization of knowledge-based tools.

SYSTEMS INTEGRATION

Many CDDSS began as research projects and are designed as stand-alone systems. Basic technical issues, such as data storage formats (a level below knowledge representation format) and communication with outside systems, often receive little attention, which can severely limit future deployment possibilities. As experience with the Arden syntax has shown,[52] even when knowledge reuse and integration are taken into account during the design stage, there is still no guarantee that these goals will be realized. At present there exists no standard for data storage and retrieval in clinical information systems. Vendors frequently consider this information proprietary and the existence of a consulting/systems integration industry which thrives on this "electronic Babel" tends to mitigate against its foreseeable demise. The inevitable deployment of electronic medical records, and the need to study clinical processes for outcomes variations assures that, unless such standards are developed and adhered to, these matters will continue to be a source of considerable consternation for all those who need support for complex decision making tasks.

CONCLUSION

The history of artificial intelligence in medicine is a mixed one of impressive creativity coupled with limited successes, small gains, and in the case of Engle,[4] cynical resignation. The various approaches taken in creating systems, while permitting narrow domain breakthroughs, all have serious limitations when attacking broad domain problems. Our incomplete understanding of the clinical reasoning process and lack of an all encompassing "theory of medicine" shall continue to be both sources of consternation and wonderfully intriguing research problems. Should research in this area continue? Of course. The work done on knowledge representation, reasoning mechanisms, machine learning, and knowledge acquisition has wide applicability and many potential benefits for society even if no robust medical expert system is ever built.

Do physicians really want help with the diagnostic process? This is a question of social and cognitive processes for which the answer to-date appears to be a very cool "perhaps". In part, the lack of acceptance may be due to physicians' limited exposure to CDDSS. The less-than-enthusiastic reception that these tools have received indicates that they also may not be addressing the perceived needs of clinicians. In addition, many current systems have serious ease-of-use problems. The final note of caution is philosophical rather than technical. Should all the problems associated with the design and implementation of CDDSS ultimately be solved, to gain wide acceptance they must provide decision support without violating two of the most fundamental social and intellectual features of the practice of medicine. First, they must not intrude on the sanctity of the patient-physician relationship. Secondly, they must do nothing to remove or alter the sheer human joy experienced in arriving at the correct diagnosis.

REFERENCES

1. Shortliffe EH. Computer-Based Medical Consultations: MYCIN. New York, NY: Elsevier Computer Science Library, Artificial Intelligence Series, 1976.

2. Weiss SM, Kulikowski CA, Amarel S et al. A model-based method for computer-aided medical decision making. Artif Intell 1978; 11:145-172.

3. de Dombal FT, Leaper DJ, Staniland JR et al. Computer aided diagnosis of acute abdominal pain. Br Med J 1972; 2:9-13.

4. Engle EL. Attempts to use computers as diagnostic aids in medical decision making: a thirty-year experience. Perspect Biol Med 1992; 35:207-219.

5. Berner ES, Webster GD, Shugerman AA et al. Performance of four computer-based diagnostic systems. N Engl J Med 1994; 330: 1792-1796.

6. Miller R, Masarie FE, Myers J. Quick Medical Reference (QMR) for diagnostic assistance. MD Comput 1986; 3:34-48.

7. Warner HR Jr. Iliad: moving medical decision-making into new frontiers. Methods Inf Med 1989; 28:370-372.

8. Barnett GO, Cimino JJ, Hupp JA et al. DXplain—an evolving diagnostic decision-support system. JAMA 1987; 258:67-74.

9. Heckerman DE, Horvitz EJ, Nathwani BN. Toward normative expert systems: Part I. The Pathfinder project. Methods Inf Med 1992; 31:90-105.

10. Shortliffe EH. The adolescence of AI in medicine:Will the field come of age in the 90s? Artif Intell Med 1993; 5:93-106.

11. Clayton PD, Hripcsak G. Decision support in healthcare. Int J Biomed Comput 1995; 39:59-66

12. Heathfield HA, Wyatt J. Philosophies for the design and development of clinical decision-support systems. Methods Inf Med 1993; 32:1-8.

13. Buchanan BG, Feigenbaum EA. Dendral and Metadendral: their applications and dimension. Artif Intell 1978; 11:5-24.

14. McDermott J. R1: A rule-based configurer of computer systems. Artif Intell 1982; 19:39-88.

15. Russell S, Norvig P. Artificial Intelligence: A Modern Approach. Upper Saddle River: Prentice-Hall, 1995.

16. Luger GF, Stubblefield WA. Artificial Intelligence and the Design of Expert Systems. Redwood City, CA: Benjamin/Cummings Publishing Company, Inc., 1989.

17. Kokol P, Mernik M, Zavrsnik J et al. Decision trees based on automatic learning and their use in cardiology. J Med Syst 1994; 18:201-206.

18. Baxt WG. Use of an artificial neural network for the diagnosis of acute myocardial infarction. Ann Intern Med 1991; 115:843-848.

19. Minsky M. A framework for representing knowledge. In: Haugeland J, ed. Mind Design. Cambridge, MA: MIT Press, 1981:95-128.
20. Pinciroli F, Combi C, Pozzi G. Object oriented DBMS techniques for time oriented medical records. Med Inf 1992; 17:231-241.
21. Frost RD, Gillenson ML. Integrated clinical decision support using an object-oriented database management system. Meth Inform Med 1993; 32:154-160.
22. Long W. Medical diagnosis using a probabilistic causal network. Appl Artif Intell 1989; 3:367-383.
23. Patil R, Szolovits P, Schwartz W. Causal understanding of patient illness and diagnosis. Proc Seventh Int Joint Conf Artif Intell 1981:893-899.
24. Allen JF. Towards a general theory of action and time. Artif Intell Med 1984; 23:123-154.
25. Sharhar Y, Musen M. A temporal-abstraction system for patient monitoring. Proc Annu Symp Comput Appl Med Care 1992: 121-127.
26. Kahn MG, Fagan LM, Sheiner LB. Model-based interpretation of time-varying medical data. Proc Annu Symp Comput Appl Med Care 1989: 28-32.
27. Kohane IS. Temporal reasoning in medical expert systems. Medinfo 1986; 5:170-174.
28. Aliferis CF, Cooper GF, Miller RA et al. A temporal analysis of QMR. JAMIA 1996; 3:79-91.
29. Reiter R. A logic for default reasoning. Artif Intell 1980; 13:81-132.
30. Patil R. Review of causal reasoning in medical diagnosis. Proc Annu Symp Comput Appl Med Care 1986:11-16.
31. Miller RA. Internist-1/Caduceus:problems facing expert consultant programs. Methods Inf Med 1984; 23:9-14.
32. Laursen P. Event detection on patient monitoring data using causal probabilistic networks. Methods Inf Med 1994; 33:111-115.
33. Rutledge GW, Andersen SK, Polaschek JX et al. A belief network model for interpretation of ICU data. Proc Annu Symp Comput Appl Med Care 1990: 785-789.
34. Pradhan M, Provan G, Henrion M. Experimental analysis of large belief networks for medical diagnosis. Proc Annu Symp Comput Appl Med Care 1994:775-779.
35. Pearl J. Probabilistic Reasoning in Intelligent Systems: Networks of Plausible Inference. San Mateo, CA: Morgan-Kaufman, 1988.
36. Sonnenberg FA, Hagerty CG, Kulikowski CA. An architecture for knowledge-based construction of decision models. Med Decis Making 1994; 14:27-39.
37. Cooper G. Probabilistic and decision-theoretic systems in medicine. Artif Intell Med 1993; 5:289-292.
38. Zadeh LA. Fuzzy logic, neural networks, and soft computing. Comm of ACM. 1994; 37:77-84.

39. Zimmerman HJ. Fuzzy Set Theory and Its Applications. 2nd ed. Amsterdam: Kluwer-Nijhoff, 1990.
40. Maiers JE. Fuzzy set theory and medicine: the first twenty years. Proc Annu Symp Comput Appl Med Care 1985:325-329.
41. Shafer G. A Mathematical Theory of Evidence. Princeton, NJ: Princeton University Press, 1976.
42. McDermott D, Doyle J. Non-monotonic logic-I. Artif Intell 1980; 13:41-72.
43. Kolodner JL, Leake DB. A tutorial introduction to case-based reasoning. In:Leake D, ed. Case-Based Reasoning: Experiences, Lessons and Future Directions. Cambridge, MA:AAAI Press/MIT Press, 1996:31-67.
44. Stamper R, Todd BS, Macpherson P. Case-based explanation for medical diagnostic programs, with an example from gynaecology. Methods Inf Med 1994; 33:205-213.
45. Koton P. Reasoning about evidence in causal explanations. Proc Seventh Nat Conf Artif Intell 1988:256-261.
46. Quinlan JR. Induction in decision trees. Machine Learning 1986; 1:81-106.
47. Su MC. Use of neural networks as medical diagnosis expert systems. Comput Biol Med 1994; 24:419-429.
48. Doyle HR, Parmanto B, Munro PW et al. Building clinical classifiers using incomplete observations—a neural network ensemble for hepatoma detection in patients with cirrhosis. Methods Inf Med 1995; 34:253-258.
49. Patil S, Henry JW, Rubenfire M et al. Neural network in the clinical diagnosis of pulmonary embolism. Chest 1993; 104:1685-1689.
50. Goldberg DE. Genetic Algorithms in Search, Optimization, and Machine Learning. Reading, MA: Addison-Wesley, 1989.
51. Weed LL. Knowledge Coupling: New Premises and New Tools for Medical Care and Education. New York, NY: Springer-Verlag, 1991.
52. Shwe M, Sujansky W, Middleton B. Reuse of knowledge represented in the Arden syntax. Proc Annu Symp Comput Appl Med Care 1992: 47-51.

$$====== \text{CHAPTER 8} ======$$

Clinical Trials of Information Interventions

E. Andrew Balas and Suzanne Austin Boren

Chapter 3 discussed the results of studies that have been conducted to determine the accuracy of clinical diagnostic decision support systems (CDDSS). When a CDDSS passes the test of accuracy and is ready for clinical implementation, the need for replicable and generalizable measurement of practical impact emerges. It is increasingly acknowledged that measurement of system performance and impact represents the research component of informatics projects and such evaluations should guide the development of decision support technologies.[1] This chapter discusses the methodology for systematic evaluation of information interventions. It provides a framework for designing appropriate tests of the clinical impact of CDDSS.

Several studies have demonstrated that computers are able to influence the behavior of providers, management of patients, and outcome of health care in many clinical areas.[2-4] Unfortunately many of the claims for computerized medical information systems seem to exceed the documented benefits. Many predictions about the computer revolution have not been realized and the evidence arising from various clinical experiments is often controversial.[5-6] There is an increasing demand to provide convincing evidence of the benefits of clinical information services.[7-8]

THE PRACTICAL AND SCIENTIFIC NEED
FOR CLINICAL TESTING

Few medical questions have been more controversial than the clinical usefulness of computer systems. Early on in the development of clinical computing applications it was suggested that the ability of computers to store information on patient history, physical findings, and laboratory data would assist in decision making, thereby freeing the physician to focus on other aspects of clinical care.[9] However, enthusiasm for the potential of the computer as an intellectual tool eroded quickly. For example, some studies indicated that a computer system for diagnosing abdominal pain generated more accurate information and reduced perforation rate.[10-11] Other studies concluded that the same system had no useful role in this diagnosis.[12-13]

Early computer system evaluations often assumed that more patient information meant better patient care. However, evaluation of techniques such as electronic fetal heart rate monitoring illustrate that this is not always the case. In the early 1970s, the common perception was that continuous heart rate monitoring can protect the fetus from prolonged intrauterine oxygen deprivation.[14-15] Subsequently, several controlled clinical trials failed to demonstrate any clinical benefit of this technology.[16-18]

Insufficient demonstration of quality improvement has been repeatedly criticized by evaluators of clinical computer applications. In a review of reports on clinical computer systems, over 75% of 135 articles were anecdotal, and only half of the remainder met basic scientific criteria for the conduct of clinical trials.[7] Piantadosi and Byar[8] concluded that a basic shift is required in how scientists view research concepts as opposed to research results; the former are generally not considered proper objects for review or dissemination. Similar issues have been raised also in other areas of health sciences. For example, Tyson et al.[19] conducted a systematic review and in only 10% of the reports were the conclusions of the investigators supported by the evidence they presented.

Some argue that medical information systems need not justify themselves in terms of improved patient outcomes because these systems are designed to influence primarily the providers of health care.[20] Therefore, only the change in the process of care has to be demonstrated (e.g., performance of clinicians). This argument is acceptable when the process of care affected has an obvious relationship to health care outcomes (e.g., certain cancer screening procedures). However, there are numerous aspects of health care for which the relationship between process and outcome is unclear (e.g., completeness of medical records).

Nevertheless, in order to compete for the resources of health care providers, system developers have to demonstrate the relevance of their computer programs to health care quality improvement and cost control. Medical practice involves a tremendous amount of information processing: collecting patient data, sharing information with patients, decision making in diagnostics and therapeutics, documenting care, communicating with other health care professionals, and educating patients. However, health care organizations invest on average only 2.6% of their operating budget in information technology, a marked contrast with the average 8-9% invested by the banking industry.[21] During the past decades, computer systems have become active ingredients of health services, but the assessment of the new information technology is still considered to be a controversial issue. Practitioners interested in applying the new information technologies need information on the results of the clinical evaluation of computer systems.

The recurrent debate over health care reform and the intensive search for cost-effective methods to improve patient care repeatedly highlight the need for adequate technology assessment of clinical information systems. Although early evaluation studies focused on the accuracy of information generated by the computer system, newer studies tend to focus on differences in the process or outcome of care due to the computer system. Although health care is clearly an information-intensive service, the clinical value of computer applications is often questioned due to the lack of demonstrated clinical benefits. As health care organizations are actively searching for opportunities to improve their information systems through purchase or development, the example set by systems on the market is very important for practical and theoretical purposes as well.

RESEARCH METHODS TO DEMONSTRATE PRACTICAL IMPACT

There is a growing demand for adequate technology assessment in the field of medical informatics.[7-8] Medical technology includes not only drugs, devices and procedures used in medical care, but also the organizational and supportive systems that provide such care. Technology assessment provides practitioners with information on alternative techniques. The pioneering report of Cochrane noted that many standard medical practices lack evidence of effectiveness.[22] Concerns of costs also stimulate efforts to assess the practical value of not only new, but also established, technologies. Some argue that the assessment of health care technologies should be an iterative process and there is a need to continuously reassess existing technologies by combining evidence from all reliable sources.[22-23]

Deming's theory of continuous quality improvement depends on understanding and revising the production processes on the basis of data about the processes themselves.[24] Likewise, quality improvement efforts in health care depend on measurable quality objectives and appropriate interventions and changes in the process. Particularly, randomized controlled trials (RCTs) have direct relevance to health care quality improvement as they become increasingly important sources of information about the clinical value of various interventions (e.g., physician and patient education,[25] interventions to promote cancer screening,[26] computerized medical records[27] and home care after hospital discharge[28]).

The concept of demonstrating quality improvement by measurements is accepted in the field of medical informatics. Clinical computer system designers often use benchmark tests, surveys and historic control comparisons to indicate the quality improvement resulting from the use of the new system. However, benchmark tests only measure the technical performance of the computer programs. They do not provide useful data on the impact of the system on either the process or outcomes of care. On the other hand, surveys of users' opinions only provide indirect information about the difference the system made in patient care.

Comparison with historical controls (before-after study) is a popular method of evaluating clinical computer applications. The fact that computer systems are often connected to a patient database further encourages the use of historical controls as a baseline for evaluation.[29] Although they may provide some useful information, analyses of databases or historical control groups of patients cannot replace planned clinical experimentation.[30] The greatest concern in using historical controls is that there may be a confounding bias introduced by the different time periods. Definitions of disease and diagnostic testing methods may change over time. In the database, data may be missing either because they were lost or not recorded. Furthermore, developing hypotheses after the collection of data often leads to unplanned multiple comparisons.[31] Excessive numbers of statistical tests can easily result in misleading statistical significance, but no practical significance.

Randomized controlled clinical studies can provide the most valid information about the efficacy of computerized information systems in patient care.[32] During the last ten years, the number of randomized controlled clinical trials testing computerized information interventions increased an average of 50% annually.[32]

A review of clinical trials of clinical decision support systems provides strong evidence that some clinical decision support systems can improve physician performance.[33] However, the majority of studies assessing patient outcomes did not demonstrate significant improvements. In addition, there have been very few controlled studies of CDDSS, which have a diagnostic, as opposed to a therapy focus.

USER SATISFACTION WITH DECISION SUPPORT SYSTEMS

Measuring and managing users' attitudes toward various aspects of information systems is an important part of making computer systems successful. No clinical computer system can be successful without gaining the support of practitioners. The primary challenge of measurement is to find an appropriate control for comparison. Ideally, satisfaction should be measured before and after the introduction of the new decision support system and there should be an improvement in users' satisfaction. However, it is often challenging to develop a generic user satisfaction instrument.

There are many complex beliefs, attitudes and behaviors influencing computer use among health care professionals. A critical success criterion for how useful information systems are is the way in which computer users react to various aspects of the system. If overall satisfaction levels are high, the user will adapt his/her activities to take advantage of the computer. The user may not cooperate and may become antagonistic toward the system if satisfaction is too low. Questionnaires or surveys are tools that can be used to assess user attitudes. The particular significance of surveys is their ability to measure the acceptance of the system and the satisfaction of the users. However, a system must be used appropriately before its impact can be accurately measured. Inattention on the part of system developers to the specific clinical needs of end users may result in system underutilization or sabotage.[34-35]

Teach and Shortliffe[36] found that physician attitudes regarding computer-based clinical decision aids and a medical computing tutorial were generally favorable. Physician expectations about the effect of computer-assisted consultation systems on medical practice were also positive, although there were considerable differences among physicians. In addition, the tutorial produced a substantial increase in knowledge about computing concepts and a significant effect on physician demands.

Decision support modules built into the Health Evaluation through Logical Processes (HELP) system are described in detail in chapter 4. HELP is a clinical information system developed at LDS Hospital that includes a computer-based patient record, alerts, reminders and other decision support aids. Gardner and Lundsgaarde[37] measured the attitudes of physicians and nurses who used the HELP system through a questionnaire with fixed-choice questions supplemented with free-text comments. The respondents did not feel that computerized decision support decreased their decision-making power, nor did they feel that expert computer systems would compromise patient privacy or lead to external monitoring. The results of the survey indicated that experience with a system was the best way to break down attitudinal barriers to the use of that system.

Although surveys and questionnaires can provide direct evidence of user attitudes toward CDDSS, they are only an indirect measure of the behavioral impact of these systems.

RANDOMIZED CONTROLLED CLINICAL TRIALS OF DECISION SUPPORT SERVICES

Because medical practice requires the efficient management of information, providing information to physicians is increasingly recognized as a clinical intervention designed to influence the process and/or outcome of patient care.[30,38] The quality of care is expected to be improved by the advanced methods of decision support. However, the benefits have to be demonstrated by appropriately controlled clinical measurements. There are many types of randomized clinical trials (e.g., parallel designs, factorial designs, cross-over trials), but the basic principles are the same: prospective and contemporaneous monitoring of the effect of a randomly allocated intervention. It is widely accepted that clinical trials represent a design superior to before-and-after studies (vulnerable to changes over time that are unrelated to the effect of the intervention) or matched control studies (a much less reliable method of obtaining comparable groups of subjects). Today, not only drugs, surgical procedures, alternative care delivery techniques but also computerized decision support services are evaluated in randomized controlled trials. For example, Pozen et al.[39] tested a predictive instrument to reduce admissions to the coronary care unit. They found that the instrument had the potential to reduce coronary care unit admissions by 250,000 for acute ischemic heart disease. Over the last ten years there has been a tremendous increase in the number of RCTs addressing clinical information interventions, including decision support systems (see Fig. 8.1).

As necessary as RCTs are, they also have limitations. RCTs can test only specific hypotheses about selected aspects of computer systems. For instance, no single RCT can answer the question as to whether an integrated hospital system is good or bad. Selected information systems can be good for certain types of patients, indifferent for others, and only potentially useful for a third group of patients. Experimental evaluations of clinical computer applications (computer-assisted services) need to identify the specific conditions to be treated, specific interventions to be tested and specific outcome variables to be measured. If this is done, the results can be specific, interpretable, and useful for practical purposes.

A surprisingly high proportion of trials are performed in outpatient facilities, particularly in primary care, while relatively few trials evaluated hospital information systems. This finding is in contrast to the large sums of money spent on information systems for inpatient care.

Although clinical trials are rapidly gaining acceptance in technology assessment, the methodology of such trials does not seem to be common knowledge. Several techniques commonly used in drug trials are irrelevant in testing computerized information interventions (e.g., blinding to the intervention, placebo), while other aspects are more critical (e.g., detailed description of sites, technical specification of intervention). The evaluated effect can be either a change in the process of care (e.g., increased or reduced use of certain drugs) or in the outcome of care (e.g., lower rate of infections). A particular

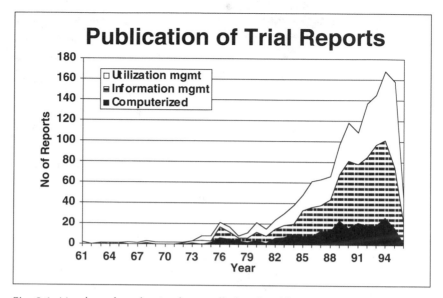

Fig. 8.1. Number of randomized controlled trials addressing clinical information interventions from 1961 to 1995.

weakness of many trials of computer systems is the lack of evaluation of patient outcome. It is certainly understandable that many information service trials evaluate the effect on care processes, since their main intent is to influence the process through the provision of accurate and timely information. However, documenting decreased side effects or other outcome measures, such as lower complication rates, could probably convince more clinicians as to their usefulness.

The setting in which the trial is conducted is critical to the representativeness of the trial. For example, the guidelines of the Nordic Council on Medicines recommend that the selection of a site for the trial has to be dependent on the potential risks involved to ensure satisfactory safety for the subjects.[40] It is a reasonable expectation that the site of a trial should represent the actual settings where the intervention will ordinarily be applied; otherwise, the generalization of the results are questionable. Many RCTs tested the effect of various interventions on the practice patterns of residents in large academic centers. It is frequently assumed that the effects will be identical when board certified physicians are subjected to the same intervention in a nonacademic environment, a hypothesis which has never been evaluated.

In health services research, randomization often assigns patients to groups through their health care providers. Major textbooks on clinical trials describe a large variety of randomization techniques.[41] However, the common feature of these techniques is that the patient is the unit of randomization. In health services research, it is often the provider who is directly targeted by the intervention. Therefore, the provider should be the unit of randomization and patients or encounters are randomized only through their providers. Our studies documented that one third of the trials on computer systems used an appropriate randomization technique.[42] The use of provider as a unit of randomization works well and could be more widely used in health services research. However, the number of providers has to be sufficient to ensure representativeness of not only the patient sample, but also of the provider sample. It is difficult to accept trials which randomize through a small number of provider units (e.g., patients of one hospital are in the study group while patients of another hospital are in the control group). In most cases, trials which randomize through less than six provider units should not be accepted as valid sources of evidence.

COLUMBIA REGISTRY OF MEDICAL MANAGEMENT TRIALS

Improving quality of care is not only a professional and ethical concern of physicians, but also the most important challenge facing a health care organization today.[24] Advanced computer techniques promise significant improvement in the quality of care through increased use of appropriate procedures and reduced use of unnecessary and potentially harmful procedures. Cochrane[43] emphasized the need to summarize evidence derived from randomized controlled trials as distinct from other kinds of evidence and to organize critical summaries by specialty or subspecialty of all relevant randomized controlled trials.

Various trial registries have been established in an attempt to improve access to published reports. Many of these registries deal with perinatal care, management for AIDS, or cancer treatment (e.g., the Oxford Perinatal Database,[44] the AIDS Clinical Trials Information Service and the National Cancer Institute (NCI) Cancer Control Intervention Studies[45]). Some review papers contain valuable bibliographies of clinical trials.[46] However clinical trials testing medical management interventions, a broad area critical to health care quality improvement and cost control, have not been the focus of any known registry.

The purpose of organizing the Columbia Registry of Medical Management Trials is to support practitioners and researchers with the best available controlled evidence on the practical value of clinical interventions changing the delivery of health services. The registry is used to facilitate access through improved MEDLINE indexing, to develop meta-analyses and reviews and to analyze the trial methodology in health services research. Examples of the interventions within the scope of our registry include patient education, reminders/prompts, feedback, computer-aided diagnosis-making and computerized records. Currently, there are approximately 1600 reports on randomized controlled clinical trials in the registry.

Specific eligibility criteria have been developed for inclusion/exclusion of reports in the Columbia Registry of Medical Management Trials. The design of the screened report is the first aspect evaluated. The study must be a prospective, contemporaneously controlled clinical trial with random assignment of intervention. Trials using allocation systems similar to a random number table (e.g., alternating encounters, alternating days of the week) are also eligible. Reports that do not meet this basic criterion (e.g., nonrandomized trial groups, review articles) are not included in the registry. Second, there should be an information management intervention in the study group with no similar intervention in the control group. Often, the control group simply receives the current standard of care, as compared with the experimental intervention used in the trial. The third criterion is that the effect of the intervention on the process and/or outcome of patient care must be measured. Planned or ongoing trials are not included in the registry because they do not meet this criterion.

The Columbia Registry of Medical Management Trials already serves as a valuable resource for information system developers and practitioners by systematically collecting and rearranging the knowledge from these trials into a format that can be used by practitioners and others making health care decisions. This knowledge engineering is accomplished in several steps. First, the trials are located by using a systematic approach, which is likely to outperform conventional searches. Each search consists of a study design concept and an intervention or effect concept. The study design concept is the same for each search and includes the following terms: random (truncated textword), group (truncated textword), random allocation (textword and MeSH), randomized controlled trial (publication type) and clinical trial (publication type). The second concept, intervention or effect, changes depending on specific interventions or effects. Subsequently, critical information is abstracted from the registered trials and the practical messages of such studies are made available to those who need them. The same executive summary can be used to implement organizational changes, further health care quality improvement, conduct meta-analyses, or write literature reviews.

Locating and registering eligible trials is an ongoing process, so the collection continues to grow. Several studies documented that regardless of the complexity of the search process, some eligible reports will remain unretrieved. Therefore, clinical trial registries grow not only through the inclusion of new publications, but also through the discovery of eligible studies published earlier. The developers of the Oxford Perinatal Database also noted that there is no "gold standard" available to judge the completeness of a registry.[44] With its growth, the Columbia Registry of Medical Management Trials aims to become an unparalleled source of high-quality clinical evidence in the areas of medical informatics and health services research.

The synthesis of trial results helps the identification of most effective information services. Table 8.1 shows the percentages of positive trials for different types of information interventions that are included in the registry.

The number of randomized controlled trials as the ultimate evidence on the practical difference made by a specific intervention is rapidly expanding. Meta-analysis is the use of statistical techniques to integrate results of separate, but similar, clinical trials. Instead of providing a qualitative assessment of a few studies, meta-analysis promises a systematic and quantitative synthesis of all available studies. Systematic collection procedures are designed to avoid the well-known deficiencies of the conventional "pick-and-choose" approach.[47]

Research synthesis of evidence from several randomized controlled clinical trials always raises the question of clinical efficacy. Vote-counting is an established method of expressing the success rate of a particular intervention.[48] When the number of successful trials is very high in a particular category, then the intervention is likely to make a difference. The particular advantage of vote-counting is that

Table 8.1. Information intervention categories

Information Intervention Category	No. of Reports (% positive)
Patient focus group	
Computer-assisted interactive patient education, instruction and therapy	19 (74)
Patient prompt/reminder	15 (80)
Patient-computer interactive information gathering	2 (100)
Provider focus group	
Provider prompt/reminder	19 (100)
Computer-assisted treatment planner	19 (79)
Provider feedback	19 (68)
Computerized medical record and information access	19 (74)
Prediction	6 (83)
Computer-assisted diagnosis	4 (50)
Total *	98 (85)

* Some reports test several interventions

information on the success or failure of the intervention is available from virtually all trial reports. Obviously, vote-counting does not consider the magnitude of effect. Primary research reports not providing enough information to calculate effect size estimates usually contain information about the direction of the effect. On the other hand, meta-analyses using the popular odds-ratio methods can specify the magnitude of the effect and are likely to discover additional categories of effective interventions.

Diversity, a frequent concern in research synthesis, can be an advantage as well as a disadvantage. Trials pooled together are always somewhat different in their sites, samples, interventions, and effect variables. A diversity of sites and samples (within the stated pooling criteria) can help document an intervention's success under a variety of circumstances. Diverse interventions can also help to reflect the natural variability of use in different health care organizations. For example, it would be unreasonable to demand separate testing of physician reminders for every single clinical procedure. Successfully applying a particular information intervention in a variety of settings and disease conditions increases the generalizability of results and the intervention's practical value.

As discussed in chapter 2, computerized decision support requires representation of clinical knowledge in Boolean production rules or other tightly organized structures (e.g., expression in probabilities, knowledge frames). To represent the data from clinical trials into a form that can be used in CDDSS requires knowledge engineering and the structuring of such evidence is becoming an important trend in knowledge engineering. As the amount of published scientific evidence grows, finding the right report is no longer sufficient. The report has to be supplemented with the abstraction of the specific information to meet the needs of clinicians, researchers and policy makers. Conventional abstracts by the investigators provide useful synopses, but often lack detail and standardization. An analysis of 150 trial reports led to the development and validation of a quality scoring system which can be used as an itemized checklist to portray the methodological quality of health services research trials.[42]

EFFECTIVE INFORMATION INTERVENTIONS

Randomized controlled trials confirm that four generic information interventions that are active components of computer systems can make a significant difference in patient care (patient education, treatment planner, physician and patient reminders).[49] To manage care and improve quality, computer systems of primary care should incorporate these effective information services.

Interactive patient education can help patients improve their health through health promotion, educational information on the management of medical conditions and computerized instruction. Seventy-four percent of the patient education studies were successful. Chapter 6 includes descriptions of some of these patient education studies.

A large number of studies employed the use of computer algorithms to assist in drug dosing decision making (e.g., aminoglycoside,[50] insulin,[51] digoxin,[2] phenytoin,[52] sodium nitroprusside,[53] lidocaine,[54] propranol[55] and amitriptyline[55]). For example, the first known trial of a decision support system compared the effect of computed digoxin dosage to that of unaided physician judgment.[2] The results indicated that the computer slightly outperformed the physician and that the correlation between predicted and measured serum digoxin concentrations was closer in the computer-assisted patient group. Overall, 79% of the computer assisted treatment planner studies were successful.

Reminders represent one of the primary techniques of delivering messages generated by clinical decision support systems. Reminder messages recommend specific action at the time of decision-making. Computers can scan each patient's record to identify tests and other procedures that are due. The main function of the computer system is the identification of eligible patients and triggering the use of a particular clinical procedure.

Several controlled experiments have demonstrated that physicians respond to computer generated reminders by performing the recommended interventions (e.g., influenza immunization, mammography). For example, patients of physicians who received reminders on the encounter forms were significantly more likely to have a mammogram ordered for them.[56] Procedures frequently targeted by the provider prompt/reminder trials included cancer screening[26,57] (stool occult blood, sigmoidoscopy, rectal examination, mammography, breast examination, Papanicolaou test, pelvic examination) and vaccinations (influenza,[58] pneumococcal,[59] tetanus[60] and infant immunizations[61]). All of the physician reminder studies and 80% of the patient reminder studies were successful.

The syntheses of trial results from the registry have already led to several practical and significant observations. For example, our meta-analysis of randomized controlled trials testing physician reminders concluded that this is a highly effective information intervention but the results vary depending on the targeted clinical procedure (e.g., cancer screening versus tetanus immunization).[62] These and other studies have demonstrated that computers can help to make patient care more consistent by reminding physicians to order or perform recommended procedures. Many systems show significant and beneficial impact in selected clinical areas, particularly health maintenance.

Obtaining good data is the basis for decision making about the value of diagnostic decision support systems. As more CDDSS reach the implementation stage, RCTs of their effectiveness as an information intervention will be possible. Registries of RCTs, such as the Columbia Registry, will be able to provide the data needed to answer questions about the value of particular CDDSS, the value of CDDSS in particular settings, and the value of CDDSS for particular purposes.

REFERENCES

1. Friedman CP. Where's the science in medical informatics? JAMIA 1995; 2:65-67.
2. Peck CC, Sheiner LB, Martin MM et al. Computer-assisted digoxin therapy. N Engl J Med 1973; 289:441-446.
3. McAlister NH, Covvey HD, Tong C et al. Randomized controlled trial of computer-assisted management of hypertension in primary care. Br Med J 1986; 293:670-674.
4. Tierney WM, Miller ME, McDonald CJ. The effect on test ordering of informing physicians of the charges for outpatient diagnostic tests. N Engl J Med 1990; 322:1499-1504.
5. Wones RG. Failure of low-cost audits with feedback to reduce laboratory test utilization. Med Care 1987; 25:78-82.
6. Wyatt J, Spiegelhalter D. Field trials of medical decision-aids: potential problems and solutions. Proc Annu Symp Comput Appl Med Care 1991:3-7.
7. Haynes RB, Walker CJ. Computer-aided quality assurance: a critical appraisal. Arch Intern Med 1987; 147:1297-1301.
8. Piantadosi S, Byar DP. A proposal for registering clinical trials. Control Clin Trials 1988; 9:82-84.
9. Gorry GA. Computer-assisted clinical decision making. Methods Inf Med 1973; 12:45.
10. de Dombal FT, Leaper DJ, Staniland JR et al. Computer aided diagnosis of acute abdominal pain. Br Med J 1972; 2:9-13.
11. McAdam WA, Brock BM, Armitage T et al. Twelve years experience of computer-aided diagnosis in a district general hospital. Ann R Coll Surg Engl 1990; 72:140-146.
12. Sutton GC. How accurate is computer-aided diagnosis? Lancet 1989; 2:905-908.
13. Paterson-Brown S, Vipond MN, Simms K et al. Clinical decision-making and laparoscopy versus computer prediction in the management of the acute abdomen. Br J Surg 1989; 76:1011-1013.
14. Gabert HA, Stenchever MA. Continuous electronic monitoring of fetal heart rate during labor. Am J Obstet Gynecol 1973; 115:919-923.
15. Paul RH, Hon EH. Clinical fetal monitoring. V. Effect on perinatal outcome. Am J Obstet Gynecol 1974; 118:529-533.
16. McDonald D, Grant A, Sheridan-Pereira M et al. The Dublin randomized controlled trial of intrapartum fetal heart rate monitoring. Am J Obstet Gynecol 1985; 152:524-539.
17. Shy KK, Luthy DA, Bennett FC et al. Effects of electronic fetal heart-rate monitoring, as compared with periodic auscultation, on the neu-

rologic development of premature infants. N Engl J Med 1990;
322:588-593.

18. Freeman R. Intrapartum fetal monitoring—a disappointing story. N
    Engl J Med 1990; 322:624-626.
19. Tyson JE, Furzan JA, Resich JS et al. An evaluation of the quality of
    therapeutic studies in perinatal medicine. J Pediatr 1983; 102:10-13.
20. Simborg DW, Whiting-O'Keefe QE. Evaluation methodology for
    ambulatory care information systems. Med Care 1982; 20:255-265.
21. Smith L. The coming health care shakeout. Fortune 1993; May
    17:70-75.
22. Cochrane AL. Effectiveness and Efficiency: Random Reflections on
    Health Services. London, England: Nuffield Provincial Hospitals Trust,
    1972.
23. Banta HD, Thacker SB. The case for reassessment of health care tech-
    nology: once is not enough. JAMA 1990; 264:235-240.
24. Berwick DM. Continuous improvement as an ideal in health care. N
    Engl J Med 1989; 320:53-56.
25. Vinicor F, Cohen SJ, Mazzuca SA et al. DIABEDS: a randomized trial
    of the effects of physician and/or patient education on diabetes pa-
    tient outcomes. J Chronic Dis 1987; 40:345-356.
26. McPhee SJ, Bird JA, Jenkins CN et al. Promoting cancer screening: a
    randomized, controlled trial of three interventions. Arch Intern Med
    1989; 149:1866-1872.
27. Tape TG, Campbell JR. Computerized medical records and preven-
    tive health care: success depends on many factors. Am J Med. 1993;
    94:619-625.
28. Melin AL, Bygren LO. Efficacy of the rehabilitation of elderly pri-
    mary health care patients after short-stay hospital treatment. Med
    Care 1992; 30:1004-1015.
29. Starmer CF, Lee KL, Harell FE et al. On the complexity of investi-
    gating chronic illness. Biometrics 1980; 36:333-335.
30. Byar DP. Why data bases should not replace randomized clinical tri-
    als. Biometrics 1980; 36:337-342.
31. Ingelfinger JA, Mosteller F, Thibodeau LA et al. Biostatistics in Clini-
    cal Medicine. New York: Macmillan, 1987.
32. Balas EA, Stockham MG, Mitchell JA et al. The Columbia registry of
    information and utilization management trials. JAMIA 1995;
    2:307-315.
33. Johnston ME, Langton KB, Haynes RB et al. Effects of computer-
    based clinical decision support systems on clinician performance and
    patient outcome:a critical appraisal of research. Ann Intern Med 1994;
    120:135-142.
34. Williams LS. Microchips versus stethoscopes: Calgary hospital, MDs
    face off over controversial computer system. Can Med Assoc J 1992;
    147:1534-1547.

35. Massaro TA. Introducing physician order entry at a major academic medical center: I. Impact on organizational culture and behavior. Acad Med 1993; 68:20-25.
36. Teach RL, Shortliffe EH. An analysis of physician attitudes regarding computer-based clinical consultation systems. Comput Biomed Res 1981; 14:542-558.
37. Gardner RM, Lundsgaarde HP. Evaluation of user acceptance of a clinical expert system. JAMIA 1994; 1:428-438.
38. Hershey CO, Porter DK, Breslau D et al. Influence of simple computerized feedback on prescription charges in an ambulatory clinic. Med Care 1986; 24:472-481.
39. Pozen MW, D'Agostino RB, Selker HP et al. A predictive instrument to improve coronary-care-unit admission practices in acute ischemic heart disease. N Engl J Med 1984; 310:1273-1278.
40. GCP: Nordic and European Guidelines. Austin: Pharmaco Dynamics Research, 1990.
41. Spilker B. Guide to Clinical Trials. New York: Raven, 1991.
42. Balas EA, Austin SM, Ewigman BG et al. Methods of randomized controlled clinical trials in health services research. Med Care 1995; 33:687-699.
43. Cochrane AL. 1931-1971, a critical review with particular reference to the medical profession. In G Teeling-Smith and N Wells, Medicine for the Year 2000. London: Office of Health Economics, 1979.
44. Chalmers I, Hetherington J, Newdick M et al. The Oxford Database of Perinatal Trials: developing a register of published reports of controlled trials. Control Clin Trials 1986; 7:306-324.
45. Dickersin K. Why register clinical trials?—Revisited. Control Clin Trials 1992; 13:170-177.
46. Davis DA, Thomson MA, Oxman AD et al. Evidence for the effectiveness of CME: a review of 50 randomized control trials. JAMA 1992; 268:1111-1117.
47. Antman EM, Lau J, Kupelnick B et al. A comparison of results of meta-analysis of randomized control trials and recommendations of clinical experts. Treatments for myocardial infarction. JAMA 1992; 268:240-248.
48. Light RJ, Smith PV. Accumulating evidence: procedures for resolving contradictions among different research studies. Harvard Educational Review 1971; 41:420-471.
49. Balas EA, Austin SM, Mitchell JA et al. The clinical value of computerized information services: a review of 98 randomized clinical trials. Arch Fam Med 1996; 5:271-278.
50. Begg EJ, Atkinson HC, Jeffery GM et al. Individualized aminoglycoside dosage based on pharmacokinetic analysis is superior to dosage based on physician intuition at achieving target plasma drug concentrations. Br J Clin Pharmac 1989; 28:137-141.

51. Chiarelli F, Tumini S, Morgese G et al. Controlled study in diabetic children comparing insulin-dosage adjustment by manual and computer algorithms. Diab Care 1990; 13:1080-1084.
52. Privitera MD, Homan RW, Ludden TM et al. Clinical utility of a Bayesian dosing program for phenytoin. Ther Drug Monit 1989; 11:285-294.
53. Reid JA, Kenny GNC. Evaluation of closed-loop control of arterial pressure after cardiopulmonary bypass. Br J Anaesth 1987; 59:247-255.
54. Rodman JH, Jelliffe RW, Kolb E et al. Clinical studies with computer-assisted initial lidocaine therapy. Arch Intern Med 1984; 144:703-709.
55. Ziegler DK, Hurwitz A, Hassanein RS et al. Migraine prophylaxis: a comparison of Propranolol and Amitriptyline. Arch Neurol 1987; 44:486-489.
56. Chambers CV, Balaban DJ, Carlson BL et al. Microcomputer-generated reminders: improving the compliance of primary care physicians with mammography screening guidelines. J Fam Pract 1989; 3:273-280.
57. Fordham D, McPhee SJ, Bird JA et al. The cancer prevention reminder system. MD Comput 1990; 7:289-295.
58. Chambers CV, Balaban DJ, Carlson BL. The effect of microcomputer-generated reminders on influenza vaccination rates in a university-based family practice center. J Am Board Fam Pract 1991; 4:19-26.
59. McDonald CJ, Hui SL, Smith DM et al. Reminders to physicians from an introspective computer medical record: a two-year randomized trial. Ann Int Med 1984; 100:130-138.
60. Ornstein SM, Garr DR, Jenkins RG et al. Computer-generated physician and patient reminders: tools to improve population adherence to selected preventive services. J Fam Pract 1991; 32:82-90.
61. Soljak MA, Handford S. Early results from the Northland immunization register. N Z Med J 1987; 100:244-246.
62. Austin SM, Balas EA, Mitchell JA et al. Effect of physician reminders on preventive care: Meta-analysis of randomized clinical trials. Proc Annu Symp Comput Appl Med Care 1994:121-124.

CHAPTER 9

Ethical and Legal Issues in Decision Support

Kenneth W. Goodman

Discrete maladies or illnesses tend to produce particular signs and symptoms. This natural correlation makes possible the process of diagnosis and prognosis. In fact, so strong is our belief in the regularity of signs and symptoms that the process has long been regarded as straightforward, if not easy: "...there is nothing remarkable," Hippocrates suggested some 2,400 years ago, "in being right in the great majority of cases in the same district, provided the physician knows the signs and can draw the correct conclusions from them".[1]

Of course, accurate diagnosis and prognosis can be quite difficult, even given the regularity of signs and symptoms. For one thing, "knowing the signs" requires a great deal of empirical knowledge and experience. For another, there is rarely a unique and isomorphic relationship between symptom and disease. Significantly, Hippocrates smuggles into his account a presumption of the very thing being described. To say that being right is unremarkable when one can draw the "correct conclusions" is to say that it is easy to be right when you know how to be right. Or, making an accurate diagnosis or prognosis is easy if one knows how to make an accurate diagnosis or prognosis!

The need to make accurate diagnoses is not based merely on the personal satisfaction that comes from being right, as gratifying as that is. It is based on the good effects that follow more frequently from accurate diagnoses than from inaccurate diagnoses. It is also based on the bad effects that error entails.

In the context of trust and vulnerability that shape patient-physician and patient-nurse encounters, there emerges an ethical imperative: to adhere to, or surpass, educational and professional standards, to monitor changes in one's domain, to know when one is out of one's depth. Decision support systems have the potential to assist physicians, but their use also entails a number of ethical concerns. In fact, this is evidence for the maturity of the science: new health technologies almost always raise ethical issues, and it should come as no surprise that clinical decision support would provide a number of challenges for those who use, or would use, computers to assist, guide or test clinical decisions. Any comprehensive treatment of computational diagnosis should include a review of ethical issues. In what follows, we identify a number of ethical issues and positions that emerge when intelligent machines are used to perform or support diagnostic functions, and we survey key legal and regulatory issues.

ETHICAL ISSUES

BACKGROUND AND CURRENT RESEARCH

It has been clear for more than a decade that health computing raises interesting and important ethical issues. In a crucial early contribution, a physician, a philosopher and a lawyer identified a series of ethical concerns, not the least of which are several surrounding the questions of who should use a "medical computer program" and under what circumstances.[2] Another early contribution emphasized the challenges raised by threats to physician autonomy.[3]

What has emerged since has been called the "Standard View" of computational diagnosis.[4] Randolph A. Miller, M.D., a key figure both in the scientific evolution of computational decision support and in scholarship on correlate ethical issues, has argued that "Limitations in man-machine interfaces, and more importantly, in automated systems' ability to represent the broad variety of concepts relevant to clinical medicine, will prevent 'human-assisted computer diagnosis' from being feasible for decades, if it is at all possible."[4] Another way of putting this is to say that computers cannot either in principle or at least for the foreseeable future supplant human decision makers. This observation entails ethical obligations, namely that computers ought not be relied on to do what humans do best, and that a "computer diagnosis" cannot as a matter of course or policy be allowed to trump a human decision or diagnosis.

Happily, the Standard View has been advanced not by those hostile to the development and use of clinical diagnostic decision support systems (CDDSS), but by leading proponents. The Standard View bespeaks a conservative and cautious approach to applications of a new technology, and as such captures important moral intuitions about technological change, risks and standards.

Interest in the three-way intersection of ethics, medicine and computing has increased significantly since initial efforts to explore these issues. On the one hand, professional societies such as the American Association for the Advancement of Science, the American College of Physicians and the American Medical Informatics Association have encouraged educational programs and other professional activities. On the other hand, the literature exploring this intersection has progressed significantly, and now includes the first book devoted to the topic.[5]

Three core areas of ethical concern have emerged in discussions of computer systems that are used to remind, consult or advise clinicians: (1) care standards; (2) appropriate use and users; and (3) professional relationships.[6]

CARE STANDARDS

We know a great deal about responsibility in medicine and nursing. For instance, we know that practitioners should generally not deceive their patients. We know that patients can be especially vulnerable, and that such vulnerability should be respected. And we know that physicians and nurses have a responsibility to do their best, irrespective of economic (dis)incentives, and that they should not attempt treatments that are beyond their training or expertise.

Learning how to meet these and other responsibilities in the context of a broad variety of social problems is arguably the leading task in bioethics. We must ask first whether computing tools help or hinder attempts to meet responsibilities, and second whether the tools impose new or special responsibilities. The overarching question may be put thus: does the new technology improve patient care? If the answer is affirmative we may suppose we have met an important responsibility. If the answer is negative, it seems clear we should not use the new technology. The problem is, we often do not know how to answer the question. That is, we are sometimes unsure whether care will be improved by the use of new technologies. If we want to meet the responsibility to avoid harm, for instance, we are impotent until we can determine the effects of the technology (see chapters 3 and 8 on evaluation of decision support systems). The upshot here is that error avoidance is an ethical imperative, both to maximize positive, short-term consequences and to ensure that, in the long run, informatics is not associated with error or carelessness or the kind of cavalier stance sometimes associated with high-tech boosterism.

The concept of error avoidance is wed to that of a standard of care. Standards evolve in the health professions because they plot the kinds of actions that are most successful in achieving certain ends. To fail to adhere to a standard is thus to increase the risk of error, at least in a mature science. Because errors or their consequences are generally regarded as harms or evils, the obligation to hew to standards is an ethical one.

But standards are empirical constructs, and so are open to revision. New evidence forces changes in standards. (This demonstrates why clinicians have an ethical obligation to monitor the scientific maturation of their disciplines by reading journals, attending conferences, etc.) To be sure, the precise content of any standard might be open to dispute. The "reasonable person" standard requires the postulation of a vague entity; this is particularly problematic when reasonable people disagree, as is often the case in medicine and nursing. A "community standard" similarly fails to identify a bright line between error and success in all circumstances in which it might be invoked. Note also that it is not always bad to forgo adherence to a practice standard—the standard will generally be invoked in ethical and legal contexts only when there is a bad outcome, or a flagrant disregard for the risk of a bad outcome. Sometimes there are good reasons to violate a standard. This demonstrates how some clinical progress is possible: if everyone in all cases stuck to a rigid standard there would be no internal evidence to support modifications of the standard. In other cases, standards are modified as a result of clinical trial findings, observational studies and serendipitous discoveries.

In the case of computer-assisted diagnoses, the challenge is perhaps best put in the form of a question: Does use of a decision support system increase the risk of error? Note in this regard the following three points. First, while accurate diagnosis is often linked to optimal treatment, this is not always the case: some patients are treated appropriately despite an inaccurate diagnosis, and some are treated incorrectly despite an accurate diagnosis. Second, one might still be able to provide an optimal treatment with a vague or imprecise diagnosis.[7] Third, computers can render diagnoses (or perform diagnosis-like functions) outside of clinical contexts, as for instance in tests for blood-borne pathogens,[8] cytology screens[9] and the like.

To ask if a computer diagnosis increases (or decreases) the risk of diagnostic or other error is in part to ask whether it will improve patient care. If the answer is that, on balance, the tool increases (the risk of) diagnostic error, then we should say it would be unethical to use it. Significantly, though, what is sought here is an empirical finding or a reasoned judgment—where such a finding is often lacking or even methodologically hard to come by; or where such a judgment is based on inadequate epistemic support, at least according to standards otherwise demanded to justify clinical decisions.

This means that we are pressed to answer an ethical question (Is it acceptable to use a decision support system?) in a context of scientific uncertainty (How accurate is the system?). Many challenges in contemporary bioethics share this feature, namely, that moral uncertainty parallels scientific or clinical ignorance.

What we generally want in such cases is a way to stimulate the appropriate use of new technologies without increasing patient risk. One approach to doing this is given the nearly oxymoronic term "progressive caution." The idea is this: "Medical informatics is, happily, here to stay, but users and society have extensive responsibilities to ensure that we use our tools appropriately. This might cause us to move more deliberately or slowly than some would like. Ethically speaking, that is just too bad."[10] Such a stance attempts the ethical optimization of decision-support use and development by encouraging expansion of the field, but with appropriate levels of scrutiny, oversight and, indeed, caution.

The moral imperative of error avoidance is, in other words, not anti-progressive. Rather, it is part of a large and public network of checks and balances that seek to optimize good outcomes by regulating conflicts between boosters and nay-sayers. The idea of progressive caution is just an attempt to capture the core values of that regulation.

It has been clear since the first efforts to address ethical issues in medical informatics that as computers help the sciences of medicine and nursing to progress, they will also contribute to changes in the standard of patient care. When that happens, however, it increases the likelihood that computer use will come to be required of clini-cians.[2] Put differently: In a comparatively short time, there has been a major shift in the availability and use of informatics tools. To the de-gree that informatics can improve the practice of the health profes-sions, there is a requirement that its tools be used.

This point is often the most disturbing for practitioners. It is troublesome that one might have an obligation to use a tool that has been presented as controversial and in need of further validation. But there is no contradiction here. In fact, it appears that the rise of medi-cal informatics parallels the emergence of other exciting and contro-versial tools, ranging from organ transplantation techniques and ad-vanced life support to laparoscopic surgical procedures and genetic testing and therapy. It is often the case in history that progress in-volves this tension. What is wanted is evidence that people of good will can both advance science and safeguard against abuses. Research studies that examine not just the accuracy of the systems, but how they are used, are crucial to collecting that evidence.

APPROPRIATE USE AND USERS

One way to abuse a tool is to use it for purposes for which it is not intended. Another is to use a tool without adequate training. A third way is to use a tool incorrectly (carelessly, sloppily, etc.) inde-pendently of other shortcomings.

There are a number of reasons why one should not use tools in unintended contexts. First, a tool designed for one purpose has a greater likelihood of not working, or not working well, for other pur-poses. To be sure, one might successfully perform an appendectomy with a kitchen knife, or dice vegetables with a scalpel, but it is bizarre to suggest that one should try either, except in an emergency. A medi-cal computer system may be used inappropriately if, for instance, it was designed for educational purposes but relied on for clinical deci-sion support; or developed for modest decision support (identifying a number of differential diagnoses) but used in such a way as to cause a practitioner to abandon a diagnosis arrived at by sound clinical methods.

In ethically optimizing the use of CDDSS, it is perhaps reassur-ing to know that we have many models and precedents. From ad-vanced life support and organ transplantation to developments in pharmacotherapy and genetics, society regularly has had to cope with technological change in the health sciences. Managing change requires that new tools are used appropriately and by adequately qualified practitioners. Education is at the core of such management.

Identifying qualifications and providing training must be key components of any movement to expand the use of decision support software. Ethical concerns arise when we are unsure of the appropriate or adequate qualifications and levels of training.[6]

The fear is that (1) a health care novice or (2) a health care professional ignorant of a system's design or capacity will use a decision support system in patient care. The reason the former is worthy of concern is that, as above, the practice of medicine and nursing remain human activities. A nonphysician or non-nurse cannot practice medicine or nursing, no matter how much computational support is available. This is also a concern in the context of consumer health informatics, or the widespread availability of online health advice to the untrained (see chapter 6). What this means is that the novice might not know when the system is in error or producing flawed output, when it is operating on insufficient information, when it is being used in a domain for which it was not designed, etc.

There are several reasons we must also focus ethical attention on the use of decision support software by computationally naive health professionals. Such professionals might not use such software to good effect (either by over- or under-estimating its abilities), might not be using it properly, or, like the novice, might not know when the system is being used in inappropriate contexts.

Such fears can be addressed by requirements that users of CDDSS have appropriate qualifications and be adequately trained in the use of the systems. Unfortunately, it is not yet clear what those qualifications should be, or how extensive a training program would be adequate. It is clear, however, that the use of diagnostic software cannot in the long run advance ethically without a better sense of where to establish guideposts for qualifications and training. This will be an increasingly important area of research in coming years.

A further ethical concern about appropriate use and users emerges from the potential to use decision support systems in contexts of practice evaluation, quality assessment, reimbursement for professional services and the like. One can imagine an insurance company or managed care organization using decision support to evaluate, or even challenge, clinical decisions. What makes such use problematic is precisely the same ensemble of concerns that led us to disdain applications in other contexts: the primacy of human cognitive expertise, uncertainty about adequate qualifications, and doubt about the consequences for improved patient care. This is not to say that a machine cannot give a correct answer in a particular case but, rather, that there are inadequate grounds to prefer machine decisions as a matter of general policy.

PROFESSIONAL RELATIONSHIPS

Many patients believe, mistakenly, that their physicians are omniscient. Many physicians believe, mistakenly, that their patients are ignoramuses. Recognition of these mistakes has led in recent years to the development of the idea of "shared decision making," namely that patients and providers are most productively seen as partners.[11] If this is so, and there is much to recommend it in many (though not all) instances, then we need to assess the effect of a third partner—the computer.

There are two overriding areas of ethical concern here. The first is that the computer will create conceptual or interpersonal distance between provider and patient. Communicating about uncertainty, especially when the stakes are high, has long been a challenge for clinicians. That a computer might be used to (help) render a diagnosis causes us to run the risk of what we will call the "computational fallacy." This is the view that what comes out of a computer is somehow more valid, accurate, or reliable than human output. Providers and patients who take such a view introduce a potentially erosive, if not destructive, element into shared decision making contexts. Anything that increases the likelihood that a patient decision or choice will be perceived as misguided or stupid adds to the problem that shared decision making was supposed to solve.

Now, it might be supposed that the physician or nurse can eliminate at least some of this tension by not disclosing to a patient that diagnostic support software was used in his or her case. But this introduces our second area of ethical concern, namely, the question whether patients should be given this information. The answer to this question must be determined against a background shaped by (1) patient sophistication and understanding of medical and statistical information and (2) clinician sophistication and understanding of communication approaches and strategies. In any case, it is inappropriate to use computer data or inferences to trump hesitant patients, or bully them into agreeing with a health professional.[12]

This point has been made most clearly in the discussion of prognostic scoring systems, or software used in critical care medicine in part to predict patient mortality. On the one hand, patients with poor prognoses might still benefit from extensive interventions, and these benefits might be important enough for the patient and/or family to seek them; on the other hand, patients with good survival odds might judge the prolongation of life to be of little value when weighed against the difficulty or burden of the extensive interventions.[13]

A related issue is likely to arise with increased frequency as patients gain access to decision support software and use it to make demands on physicians, or at least to challenge or second-guess them. The difficulties raised by these demands and challenges will multiply as diagnostic systems improve. As discussed in chapter 6, there is a sense in which one might regard such access as an important tool in the process of shared decision making: it will not do to expect patients to become involved in their own care and simultaneously constrain their sources of information. Contrarily, a patient might constitute a paradigm case of an inappropriate diagnostic system user, especially in those cases in which the system causes someone to forgo appropriate medical care.

We might compare patient use of diagnostic machines to patient use of medical texts and journals. In years past, there was an inclination to regard such access as risky and hence inappropriate. While a little knowledge can be dangerous, a position that does not go beyond such a view seems to miss an opportunity to educate patients about their illnesses and the relation between medical literature on the one hand and medical knowledge and practice on the other. Much the same point can be made about patient use of diagnostic tools: a physician should respond to such use by making clear that computers are not surrogates for health professionals, and that the practice of medicine entails far more than statistical induction from signs, symptoms and lab values. To be sure, it would be well if the physician's actual practice embodied this insight.

As long as the healing professions are practiced in a matrix of scientific uncertainty and patient values, we err if we appoint computational decision support as a surrogate for compassionate communication, shared decisions, and quality care by competent humans.

LEGAL AND REGULATORY ISSUES

Computers and software raise conceptually fascinating and important practical questions about responsibility and liability. Further, the question whether a decision support system is a medical device needing governmental regulation is a source of tension and debate. In both domains, scientists, clinicians, philosophers, lawyers and government and policy officials must grapple with a variety of knotty problems.

The intersection of medicine, computational decision support and law has been addressed mostly in speculative terms. The use of decision support systems is not widespread enough to have stimulated legislation or illuminating precedent. Moreover, medicine and computing share little in the way of a common legal history. The following observation is as apt today as it was more than a decade ago:

> "The introduction of computerized decision-making will require the merger of computer science and medical care; two areas with fundamentally different legal traditions. The legal differences between the computer field and medicine are striking. Medicine is tightly regulated at all levels. Most health care providers are licensed, and a rigid hierarchical system is the norm. Yet, computer systems and companies are created in a totally unregulated competitive environment in which "software piracy" is common, standardization is in its infancy, licensing is a method of transferring trade secret software, and companies begin in garages."[14]

LIABILITY AND DECISION SUPPORT

The overriding legal issue related to computational decision support is liability for use, misuse—or even lack of use—of a computer to make or assist in rendering diagnoses.[15-18] In the United States, tort law holds providers of goods and services accountable for injuries sustained by users. Because of legal and regulatory variation, there are similarities and differences in other countries.[19-21] Such accountability is addressed by either the negligence standard or the strict liability standard.

The negligence standard applies to services, and strict liability applies to goods or products, although negligence can sometimes also apply to goods, as in cases of negligent product design. There is no consensus about whether decision support systems are services or products, in part because these systems have properties that resemble both services and products.[2,14-15,22-23] For instance, a physician's diagnosis is clearly a service and any liability for erroneous diagnoses is judged by the negligence standard. If a human diagnosis is considered a service, then, it is argued, a computer diagnosis (or the task of writing the computer code that rendered the diagnosis) should have the same status. Contrarily, commercial CDDSS are manufactured, mass-marketed, and sold like entities uncontroversially regarded to be products.

An additional complication is that these systems are sold to hospitals, physicians, patients and others, and, indeed, are now available on the World Wide Web. If a patient is injured by a defective system, it remains to be determined who used the system (the physician? the patient?) and whether it was misused. Also, it can be exquisitely difficult to identify the defect in a computer program,[15] as well as to answer the important question as to whether a physician could have intervened and prevented the application of mistaken advice.[2]

Neither is there a clear standard of care for use of decision support software by clinicians. Physicians or nurses might someday be found negligent either for accepting a mistaken computer diagnosis or, having erred in diagnosis themselves, for failing to have used a decision support system that might have proved corrective. In either case, the determination of negligence will have to be weighed against prevailing community or reasonable-person standards. As with other areas of practice, errors will increase liability accordingly as the practitioner is seen to have fallen behind, or moved too far ahead of, such standards.

There is a clear need for additional conceptual analysis to assist the law in sorting out these puzzles. Local trial courts and juries will often be out of their depth if called on to adjudicate liability claims that challenge fundamental conceptions of responsibility, accountability and blame. Similar difficulties arise in other areas, such as in the intellectual property arena, when there is a need to determine whether computer software is an invention or a work of art. In one interesting approach to these questions, Professor John Snapper attempts an account of responsibility that will not impede the future— and presumably salutary—development of mechanical decision support. On this account, the attribution of responsibility and duty to computers for certain actions will maximize the good that will result from increased use of improved decision support systems.[24] The idea is that use of conceptually inadequate legal tools to punish system designers, owners and users might have a chilling effect on the evolution of decision support technology. Spreading responsibility around, and including computers as agents to which responsibility may be assigned, is said to offer the potential of stimulating system design and the benefits this would entail.

This much is clear: physicians and nurses who revile and disdain computers will be ignorant of machines that can in principle improve their practice, and hence patient care. Zealots who take computers to constitute adequate or even superior human surrogates will have lost touch with the human foundations of their profession. At either extreme the risk is high of falling outside emerging standards. This is a mistake—in ethics and at law.

REGULATION OF DECISION-SUPPORT SOFTWARE

While the history of governmental regulation of health care products is traceable to the Pure Food and Drug Acts of 1906, the regulation of medical devices was not formalized until the Federal Food, Drug, and Cosmetic Act of 1938. There, a medical device was defined as "instruments, apparatus, and contrivances, including their components, parts and accessories, intended: (1) for use in diagnosis, cure, mitigation, treatment, or prevention of diseases in man or other animals; or (2) to affect the structure or any function of the body of man or other animals."[25-26] In 1976, motivated by the increased complexity of devices and by reports of some devices' shortcomings and failures, Congress approved comprehensive Medical Device Amendments to the 1938 regulations; the amendments were to "ensure that new devices were safe and effective before they were marketed."[27-28] In 1990, a new regulation replaced that emphasis on premarket approvals with an emphasis on postmarket surveillance.[29] Proposals to regulate diagnostic software have been evaluated against the 1976 and 1990 laws and a broad array of draft policies and statements.

The U.S. Food and Drug Administration (FDA) unequivocally regards medical software as a device. The FDA identifies four types of devices:

1. Educational and Bibliographic Software
Federal authorities regard the following as exempt, or not falling under existing regulation:

- Software intended only for use in performing traditional "library" functions, such as storage, retrieval and dissemination of medical information (i.e., functions that are traditionally carried out using medical textbooks and journals).
- Software intended only for use as general accounting or communications functions.
- Software solely intended for educational purposes rather than to diagnose or treat patients.[30]

2. Software Components

Some software is incorporated into medical devices and is actively regulated. Examples include the software in:
- infusion pumps
- pacemakers
- ventilators
- magnetic resonance imaging devices
- diagnostic x-ray systems
- clinical laboratory instruments
- blood grouping instruments.[30]

3. Software Accessories

Software accessories are attached to or used with other devices, and as such are also actively regulated. These include software for:
- radiation treatment planning
- conversion of pacemaker telemetry data
- conversion, transmission or storage of medical images
- off-line analysis of EEG data
- digital analysis and graphical presentation of EEG data
- calculation of rate response for a cardiac pacemaker
- perfusion calculations for cardiopulmonary bypass
- calculation of bone fracture risk from bone densitometry data
- statistical analysis of pulse oximetry data
- calculation of refractive power of intraocular lenses[30]

4. Stand-Alone Software

The most controversial class, stand-alone software, includes CDDSS and other decision support systems. Whether such systems should be regulated is a matter of continuing debate. Examples include:

- blood bank software systems which control donor deferrals and release of blood products
- software designed to assist a health care practitioner in arriving at a diagnosis of a particular patient
- software which analyzes for potential therapeutic interventions for a particular patient
- software which records medical information for later recall, analysis, or action by a health care practitioner (e.g., hospital information systems, prescription ordering and drug interaction information systems, emergency room triage software, and various calculators which automate calculations of drug doses)[30]

In 1989, an FDA draft policy proposed regulatory exemption for "Previously unclassified information management products ... such as expert or knowledge based systems, artificial intelligence and other types of decision support systems intended to involve competent human intervention before any impact on human health occurs."[31] The question then became whether CDDSS were intended to involve competent human intervention. The FDA is currently reconsidering this regulatory exemption. In chapter 1, Miller and Geissbuhler examine some of the issues connected with FDA regulation.

While the FDA regards software as a device, there are a number of reasons why it might be best if medical decision support software were not subjected to thorough federal regulation. The most common arguments against regulation include the following:

- Software is most accurately regarded as a mental construct or abstract entity, i.e., the sort of thing not customarily falling within the FDA's regulatory purview.
- Practitioners—not software—have traditionally been subjected to licensing requirements.
- Software evolves rapidly and locally, and any sort of national software monitoring is likely to be ineffective or impossible.
- Software is imperfect, and so improvement and refinement—not perfection—must be the standard to be striven for and met. Yet at law, strict liability standards (usually applied to devices or goods but not services) require perfection.

Several of these points could be in line with an influential stance held by a former commissioner of the agency, namely that the FDA should "apply the least regulation allowed to remain consistent with the requirements of public health and safety."[32]

The debate over medical software regulation represents one of the most important controversies of the Computer Age. The balancing of risks and benefits, as well as public safety and technological progress, means that scientists, clinicians and policy makers have one of civilization's most interesting—and challenging—tasks.

CONCLUSION AND FUTURE DIRECTIONS

Clinicians, philosophers, lawyers and policy makers have grappled for more than a decade with social, ethical and legal issues raised by the growth of health informatics, perhaps especially by progress in development of tools for computational diagnosis. What has emerged is a recognition that future scientific growth must be guided by corresponding attention to ethical issues. These issues address the role of error avoidance and standards; of appropriate use and users; and of professional relationships. Scientific programs and publications may be regarded as duty-bound to foster environments in which further attention to ethical, legal and social issues is encouraged. Indeed, to the extent that morality guides the law, vigorous programs to identify and debate ethical issues will be of no small service to society as legislatures, courts and government regulators and policy makers attempt to apply the insights of ethics to practical problems in health informatics.

More research on ethical issues in computational diagnosis is essential for this process. We have, for instance, only begun to address issues that arise when diagnostic tools are made available on the World Wide Web; we are in no way clear about the level of ethics education that is appropriate for students in health informatics; and there is much work to be done at the intersections of ethics and system evaluation and ethics and standards of care.

Elsewhere in the history of science and technology, such challenges are often taken to constitute evidence of the growth and maturation of an applied science. This is no less true for computational diagnosis and, indeed, for all of health informatics.

References

1. Hippocrates. Prognosis. In Lloyd GER, ed. Hippocratic Writings, translated by Chadwick J, Mann WN. London: Penguin Books 1983:170-185.
2. Miller RA, Schaffner KF, Meisel A. Ethical and legal issues related to the use of computer programs in clinical medicine. Ann Intern Med 1985; 102:529-536.
3. de Dombal FT. Ethical considerations concerning computers in medicine in the 1980s. J Med Ethics 1987; 13:179-184.
4. Miller RA. Why the standard view is standard: people, not machines, understand patients' problems. J Med Philos 1990; 15:581-591.
5. Goodman KW, ed. Ethics, Computing and Medicine: Informatics and the Transformation of Health Care. Cambridge and New York: Cambridge University Press, 1997.
6. Miller RA, Goodman KW. Ethical challenges in the use of decision-support software in clinical practice. In: Goodman KW, ed. Ethics, Computing and Medicine: Informatics and the Transformation of Health Care. Cambridge and New York: Cambridge University Press, 1997:102-115.
7. Berner ES, Webster GD, Shugerman AA et al. Performance of four computer-based diagnostic systems. N Engl J Med 1994; 330: 1792-1796.
8. Sorace JM, Berman JJ, Carnahan GE et al. PRELOG: precedence logic inference software for blood donor deferral. Proc Annu Symp Comput Appl Med Care 1991: 976-977.
9. Boon ME, Kok LP. Neural network processing can provide means to catch errors that slip through human screening of Pap smears. Diag Cytopath 1993; 9:411-416.
10. Goodman KW. Bioethics and health informatics: an introduction. In: Goodman KW, ed. Ethics, Computing and Medicine: Informatics and the Transformation of Health Care. Cambridge and New York: Cambridge University Press, 1997:1-31.
11. Forrow L, Wartman SA, Brock DW. Science, ethics, and the making of clinical decisions. JAMA 1988; 259:3161-3167.
12. Goodman KW. Outcomes, futility, and health policy research. In: Goodman KW, ed. Ethics, Computing and Medicine: Informatics and the Transformation of Health Care. Cambridge and New York: Cambridge University Press, 1997:116-138.
13. Brody BA. The ethics of using ICU scoring systems in individual patient management. Prob Crit Care 1989; 3:662-670.
14. Brannigan VM, Dayhoff RE. Medical informatics: the revolution in law, technology, and medicine. J Legal Med 1986; 7:1-53.
15. Miller RA. Legal issues related to medical decision-support systems. Int J Clin Monit Comput 1989; 6:75-80.
16. Mortimer H. Computer-aided medicine: present and future issues of liability. Computer Law J 1989; 9:177-203.

17. Turley TM. Expert software systems: the legal implications. Computer Law J 1988; 8:455-477.
18. Hafner AW, Filipowicz AB, Whitely WP. Computers in medicine: liability issues for physicians. Int J Clin Monit Comput 1989; 6:185-194.
19. Beier B. Liability and responsibility for clinical software in the Federal Republic of Germany. Comput Methods Programs Biomed 1987; 25:237-242.
20. Brahams D, Wyatt J. Decision aids and the law. Lancet 1918; ii:632-634.
21. Allaërt FA, Dussere L. Decision support system and medical liability. Proc Annu Symp Comput Appl Med Care 1992:750-753.
22. Birnbaum LN. Strict products liability and computer software. Computer Law J 1988; 8:135-156.
23. Gill CJ. Medical expert systems: grappling with the issues of liability. High Tech Law J 1987; 1:483-520.
24. Snapper JW. Responsibility for computer-based decisions in health care. In: Goodman KW, ed. Ethics, Computing and Medicine: Informatics and the Transformation of Health Care. Cambridge and New York: Cambridge University Press, 1997, 43-56.
25. Munsey RR. Trends and Events in FDA regulation of medical devices over the last fifty years. Food and Drug Law J 1995; 50:163-177.
26. Public Law No. 75-717, 52 Stat. 1040 (1938), as amended 21 U.S.C. Sections 301 et seq (1988).
27. Kessler DA, Pape SM, Sundwall DN. The federal regulation of medical devices. N Engl J Med 1987; 317:357-366.
28. Public Law No. 94-295, 90 Stat. 539 (1976), codified at 21 U.S.C. Sections 360c et seq (1982).
29. Brannigan VM. Software quality regulation under the Safe Medical Devices Act of 1990: hospitals are now the canaries in the software mine. Proc Annu Symp Comput Appl Med Care 1991:238-242.
30. Food and Drug Administration. FDA regulation of medical device software. (Document prepared for an FDA Software Policy Workshop, Sept. 3-4, 1996, National Institutes of Health, Bethesda, Md.). http://www.fda.gov//cdrh/ost/points.html.
31. Food and Drug Administration, Center for Devices and Radiological Health. Policy for the Regulation of Computer Products, draft, 13 November 1989. Rockville, Maryland: FDA, CDRH, 1989.
32. Young FE. Validation of medical software: present policy of the Food and Drug Administration. Ann Intern Med 1987; 106:628-629.

This book has examined a range of clinical diagnostic decision support systems (CDDSS) that are currently available for clinicians, for students, and for patients and has shown the potential that these systems have to influence both patient health outcomes and the cost of medical care. It is likely that new CDDSS will become available, some of the CDDSS described in this book will improve and adapt to new modes of delivery and others may become obsolete. We have also discussed some of the obstacles to future development that must be overcome if these systems are to realize their potential, as well as the ethical concerns that must accompany future development and implementation of CDDSS. That there will be continued development of CDDSS is a given, but when these systems will be mature enough to be routinely available is not yet known. Not only are there technical issues that must be addressed, but there are changes in attitudes that must also occur.

When I have given talks on CDDSS to physicians and others outside the medical informatics community, the audience often reacts very strongly, yet the concerns expressed are almost contradictory. In response to hearing that CDDSS provide information for the physician to consider, rather than generating a single correct answer, there are responses such as, "What use are they if they don't give the answer?" or " There is no way physicians will document in their records that they used a system that might be wrong." At the same time, there are concerns expressed that a physician who needs or benefits from a CDDSS is somehow "not expert enough" to be a "good doctor." Even the contributors to this book, who are specialists in medical informatics and who are very well-versed in the nuances of the CDDSS described, differ in their attitudes regarding the likely impact of these programs. Probably all of them are cautiously optimistic about the future of these systems, but some are more optimistic, and others lean more to the side of caution.

To put the role of CDDSS in perspective, it might be helpful to consider an analogy to the use of a spell checker in a word processor. The spell checker alerts the user of the word processor to possible spelling errors which the user must verify. Anyone who has used these systems has seen the often amusing "incorrect" suggestions that these systems produce. The user needs enough spelling knowledge to be able to determine if the spell-checker is correct, but clearly benefits from the alerts, *even if many of them must be disregarded.* Because it is assumed that the user has more, or better, information than the system, it is taken for granted that the user can benefit from the use of the spell checker and can ignore the erroneous suggestions.

Because general computer-based tools are now routinely available, word processor users are not considered more of an "expert" speller if they do not use the spell-checker. Rather, they are seen as careless if they produce a document with errors because they failed to use the system, and they would be considered inefficient if they refused to use it because they preferred to check the entire document by themselves without it. Clearly in the latter case, there is also a greater possibility for error.

The process of medical diagnosis is obviously more complex than spelling, which is one reason why spell-checkers are ubiquitous today and CDDSS are not. But even when CDDSS are more widely available, for them to be used appropriately we may have to change our thinking regarding what it means to be an "expert" diagnostician. As repeatedly stressed throughout this book, a CDDSS will be very unlikely to function as an expert, independent of the clinician. Yet, CDDSS are going to continue to improve, they will become linked to and incorporated into other computer-based systems, and they will be more readily accessible to support clinicians. When that occurs and they become more widely utilized, the term "expert system" may again be appropriate to use; however, when that time comes, the emphasis will be on the word system, to refer to the human-computer combination. Clinicians who feel that they do not need this support may be seen, not as the more trusted expert, but as foolishly subjecting their patients to potential diagnostic error. And we will recognize the true "experts" as the health professionals who understand the limits of these tools, who have the knowledge to recognize when the computers are providing useful information, and who have the expertise to use them to enhance their diagnostic performance, and perhaps, even their own cognition.

═══════════════ APPENDIX ═══════════════

EXAMPLES OF INTERNET RESOURCES FOR PATIENTS*

AHCPR Consumer Health Information - Agency for Health Care Policy and Research site with consumer information - http://www.ahcpr.gov/clinic/

AHCPR Practice Guidelines and Medical Outcomes - http://gopher.nlm.gov:80/guide/

American Cancer Society - patient information - http://www.cancer.org/cancinfo.html

CancerNet - Information for Patients - detailed information for both physicians and consumers - cancernet.nci.nih.gov/patient.html

National Council for Reliable Health Informaton (Reuters Health Information Service) http://www.ncahf.org

HealthWeb - Consumer health information from University of Illinois at Chicago Health Sciences Library - http://www.uic.edu/depts/lib/health/hw/consumer/

IPDG Consumer Health Information Resources - http://www.ohsu.edu/bicc-ipdg

Medical Matrix/Patient Education - General resource for patient education sites on the Internet - http://www.medmatrix.org/SPages/Patient_Education.asp

Netwellness™ - An electronic health library - http://www.netwellness.com

The Health Explorer - Consumer health information database - http://www.healthexplorer.com/text/

Newsletters on the Internet:

Harvard Health Newsletters www.countway.med.harvard.edu/publications/Health_Publications/index.html

Mayo Clinic - http://www.mayo.ivi.com/ivi/mayo/common/htm/index.htm

The Medical Reporter - http://www.dash.com/netro/nwx/tmr/tmr.html

ONCOLINK - The University of Pennsylvania Cancer Resource - A comprehensive site for information on both adult and pediatric cancer - http://oncolink.com

PharmInfoNet - Pharmaceutical Information Network and Drug database - http://pharminfo.org

Put Prevention into Practice - Department of Health and Human Services site - http://odphp.oash.dhhs.gov/

The Virtual Hospital - University of Iowa Information for Patients - http://indy.radiology.uiowa.edu/Patients/Patients.html

*Sites listed were current at time of publication.

REFERENCES

Adams ID, Chan M, Clifford PC et al. Computer aided diagnosis of acute abdominal pain: a multicentre study. Br Med J (Clin Res Ed) 1986; 293:800-804.

Aliferis CF, Cooper GF, Miller RA et al. A temporal analysis of QMR. JAMIA 1996; 3:79-91.

Aliferis CF, Miller RA. On the heuristic nature of medical decision-support systems. Methods Inf Med 1995; 34:5-14.

Allaërt FA, Dussere L. Decision support system and medical liability. Proc Annu Symp Comput Appl Med Care 1992:750-753.

Allen JF. Towards a general theory of action and time. Artif Intell Med 1984; 23:123-154.

Allen JK, Becker DM, Swank RT. Factors related to functional status after coronary artery bypass surgery. Heart Lung 1990; 19:337-343.

Alterman AI, Baughman TG. Videotape versus computer interactive education in alcoholic and nonalcoholic controls. Alcoholism 1991; 15:39-44.

Anderson RE, Hill RB, Key CR. The sensitivity and specificity of clinical diagnostics during five decades. JAMA 1989; 261:1610-1617.

Anderson RM, Funnell MM, Butler PM et al Patient empowerment. Results of a randomized trial. Diabetes Care 1995; 18:943-949.

Antman EM, Lau J, Kupelnick B et al. A comparison of results of meta-analysis of randomized control trials and recommendations of clinical experts. Treatments for myocardial infarction. JAMA 1992; 268:240-248.

Astion ML, Wener MH, Thomas RG et al. Application of neural networks to the classification of giant cell arteritis. Arthritis Rheum 1994; 37:760-770.

Austin SM, Balas EA, Mitchell JA et al. Effect of physician reminders on preventive care: Meta-analysis of randomized clinical trials. Proc Annu Symp Comput Appl Med Care 1994:121-124.

Bacchus CM, Quinton C, O'Rourke K et al. A ramdomized crossover trial of quick medical reference (QMR) as a teaching tool for medical interns. J Gen Intern Med 1994; 9:616-621.

Balas EA, Austin SM, Ewigman BG et al. Methods of randomized controlled clinical trials in health services research. Med Care 1995; 33:687-699.

Balas EA, Austin SM, Mitchell JA et al. The clinical value of computerized information services: a review of 98 randomized clinical trials. Arch Fam Med 1996; 5:271-278.

Balas EA, Stockham MG, Mitchell JA et al. The Columbia registry of information and utilization management trials. JAMIA 1995; 2:307-315.

Bandura A. Human agency in social cognitive theory. Am Psychol 1989; 44:1175-1184.

Bandura A. Self-efficacy: towards a unifying theory of behavioral change. Psychol Rev 1977; 84:191-215.

Bankowitz RA. The effectiveness of QMR in medical decision support. Executive summary and final report. Springfield, VA: U.S. Department of Commerce, National Technical Information Service, 1994.

Bankowitz RA, Lave JR, McNeil MA. A method for assessing the impact of a computer-based decision support system on health care outcomes. Methods Inf Med 1992; 31:3-11.

Bankowitz RA, McNeil MA, Challinor SM et al. A computer-assisted medical diagnostic consultation service: implementation and prospective evaluation of a prototype. Ann Intern Med 1989; 110:824-832.

Bankowitz RA, McNeil MA, Challinor SM et al. Effect of a computer-assisted general medicine diagnostic consultation service on housestaff diagnostic strategy. Methods Inf Med 1989; 28:352-356.

Banta HD, Thacker SB. The case for reassessment of health care technology: once is not enough. JAMA 1990; 264:235-240.

Bar-Hillel M. The base-rate fallacy in probability judgments. Acta Psychol 1980; 44:211-233.

Barness LA, Tunnessen WW Jr, Worley WE et al. Computer-assisted diagnosis in pediatrics. Am J Dis Child 1974; 127:852-858.

Barnett GO, Cimino JJ, Hupp JA et al. DXplain—an evolving diagnostic decision-support system. JAMA 1987; 258:67-74.

Barnett GO, Hoffer EP, Packer MS et al. DXplain—demonstration and discussion of a diagnostic decision support system. Proc Annu Symp Comput Appl Med Care 1992:822.

Barnett GO. Information technology and medical education at Harvard Medical School. In: R. Salamon R, Protti D, Moehr J, eds. Proceedings Medical Informatics & Education International Symposium. Victoria B.C.:International Medical Informatics Association, 1989:3-5.

Barnett GO. Information technology and medical education. JAMIA 1995; 2:285-291.

Barrows HS, Norman GR, Neufeld VR et al. The clinical reasoning of randomly selected physicians in general medical practice. Clin Invest Med 1982; 5:49-55.

Baxt WG. A neural network trained to identify the presence of myocardial infarction bases some decisions on clinical associations that differ from accepted clinical teaching. Med Decis Making 1994; 14:217-222.

Baxt WG. Use of an artificial neural network for the diagnosis of acute myocardial infarction. Ann Intern Med 1991; 115:843-848.

Bayes T. An essay towards solving a problem in the doctrine of chances. Philosophical Transactions 1763; 3:370-418.

Beck JR, O'Donnell JF, Hirai F et al. Computer-based exercises in anemia diagnosis (PlanAlyzer). Methods Inf Med 1989; 28:364-369.

Begg EJ, Atkinson HC, Jeffery GM et al. Individualized aminoglycoside dosage based on pharmacokinetic analysis is superior to dosage based on physician intuition at achieving target plasma drug concentrations. Br J Clin Pharmac 1989; 28:137-141.

Behrman RE, Kliegman RM, Arvin AM, eds. Nelson Textbook of Pediatrics, 15th ed. Philadelphia: W.B. Saunders Company, 1996.

Beier B. Liability and responsibility for clinical software in the Federal Republic of Germany. Comput Methods Programs Biomed 1987; 25:237-242.

Beisecker AE, Beisecker TD. Patient information-seeking behaviors when communicating with doctors. Med Care 1990; 28:19-28.

Berman L, Miller RA. Problem area formation as an element of computer aided diagnosis: a comparison of two strategies within quick medical reference (QMR). Methods Inf Med 1991; 30:90-95.

Berner ES. The problem with software reviews of decision support systems. MD Comput 1993; 10:8-12.

Berner ES, Maisiak RS. Physician use of interactive functions in diagnostic decision support systems. Proc AMIA Fall Symp 1997, 842.

Berner ES, Jackson JR, Algina J. Relationships among performance scores of four diagnostic decision support systems. JAMIA 1996; 3:208-215.

Berner ES, Webster GD, Shugerman AA et al. Performance of four computer-based diagnostic systems. N Engl J Med 1994; 330:1792-1796.

Berwick DM. Continuous improvement as an ideal in health care. N Engl J Med 1989; 320:53-56.

Birnbaum LN. Strict products liability and computer software. Computer Law J 1988; 8:135-156.

Bleich HL. Computer evaluation of acid-base disorders. J Clin Invest 1969; 48:1689-1696.

Bleich HL. The computer as a consultant. N Engl J Med 1971; 284:141-146.

Blois MS, Tuttle MS, Sherertz DD. RECONSIDER: A program for generating differential diagnoses. Proc Annu Symp Comput Appl Med Care 1981:263-268.

Blois MS. Clinical judgment and computers. N Engl J Med 1980; 303:192-197.

Boon ME, Kok LP. Neural network processing can provide means to catch errors that slip through human screening of Pap smears. Diag Cytopath 1993; 9:411-416.

Bouhaddou O, Lambert JG, Morgan GE. Illiad and Medical HouseCall: evaluating the impact of common sense knowledge on the diagnostic accuracy of a medical expert system. Proc Annu Symp Comput Appl Med Care 1995:742-746.

Bouhaddou O, Warner H. An interactive patient information and education system (Medical HouseCall) based on a physician expert system (Illiad). MedInfo 1995; 0 Pt 2.1181-1185.

Bradshaw KE, Gardner RM, Pryor TA. Development of a computerized laboratory alerting system. Comput Biomed Res 1989; 22:575-587.

Brahams D, Wyatt J. Decision aids and the law. Lancet 1918; ii:632-634.

Brannigan VM. Software quality regulation under the Safe Medical Devices Act of 1990: hospitals are now the canaries in the software mine. Proc Annu Symp Comput Appl Med Care 1991:238-242.

Brannigan VM, Dayhoff RE. Medical informatics: the revolution in law, technology, and medicine. J Legal Med 1986; 7:1-53.

Brimberry R. Vaccination of high-risk patients for influenza. A comparison of telephone and mail reminder methods. J Fam Pract 1988; 26:397-400.

Brody BA. The ethics of using ICU scoring systems in individual patient management. Prob Crit Care 1989; 3:662-670.

Brody DS. The patient's role in clinical decision making. Ann Intern Med 1980; 93:718-722.

Brody DS, Miller SM, Lerman CE et al. The relationship between patients' satisfaction with their physicians and perceptions about interventions they desired and received. Med Care 1989; 27:1027-1035.

Brody DS, Miller SM, Lerman CE et al. Patient perception of involvement in medical care: relationship to illness attitudes and outcomes. J Gen Intern Med 1989; 4:506-511.

Brown MS. Polish and glitz aside, net resources fall short on the content yardstick. Medicine on the Net 1996; 2:7-8.

Brunswik E. Representative design and probabilistic theory in a functional psychology. Psychol Rev 1955; 62:193-217.

Buchanan BG, Feigenbaum EA. Dendral and Metadendral: their applications and dimension. Artif Intell 1978; 11:5-24.

Byar DP. Why data bases should not replace randomized clinical trials. Biometrics 1980; 36:337-342.

Cassileth B, Aupkis R, Sutton-Smith K et al. Information and participation preferences among cancer patients. Ann Intern Med 1980; 92:832-836.

Campbell DS, Neill J, Dudley P. Computer-aided self-instruction training with hearing-impaired impulsive students. Am Ann Deaf 1989; 134:227-231.

Chalmers I, Hetherington J, Newdick M et al. The Oxford Database of Perinatal Trials: developing a register of published reports of controlled trials. Control Clin Trials 1986; 7:306-324.

Chalmers TC, Smith H, Blackburn B et al. A method for assessing the quality of a randomized control trial. Control Clin Trials 1981; 2:31-49.

Chambers CV, Balaban DJ, Carlson BL et al. Microcomputer-generated reminders: improving the compliance of primary care physicians with mammography screening guidelines. J Fam Pract 1989; 3:273-280.

Chambers CV, Balaban DJ, Carlson BL. The effect of microcomputer-generated reminders on influenza vaccination rates in a university-based family practice center. J Am Board Fam Pract 1991; 4:19-26.

Chan CW, Witherspoon JM. Health risk appraisal modifies cigarette smoking behavior among college students. J Gen Intern Med 1988; 3:555-559.

Chiarelli F, Tumini S, Morgese G et al. Controlled study in diabetic children comparing insulin-dosage adjustment by manual and computer algorithms. Diab Care 1990; 13:1080-1084.

Chimowitz MI, Logigian EL, Caplan LR. The accuracy of bedside neurological diagnoses. Ann Neurol 1990; 28:78-87.

Classen DC, Pestotnik SL, Evans RS et al. Adverse drug events in hospitalized patients: excess length of stay, extra costs, and attributable mortality. JAMA 1997; 277:301-306.

Classen DC, Pestotnik SL, Evans RS et al. Computerized surveillance of adverse drug events in hospital patients. JAMA 1991; 266:2847-2851.

Clayton PD, Hripcsak G. Decision support in healthcare. Int J Biomed Comput 1995; 39:59-66.

Clayton PD, Sideli RV, Sengupta S. Open architecture and integrated information at Columbia-Presbyterian Medical Center. MD Comput 1992; 9:297-303.

Cochrane AL. 1931-1971, a critical review with particular reference to the medical profession. In G Teeling-Smith and N Wells, Medicine for the Year 2000. London: Office of Health Economics, 1979.

Cochrane AL. Effectiveness and Efficiency: Random Reflections on Health Services. London, England: Nuffield Provincial Hospitals Trust, 1972.

Console L, Molino G, Ripa di Meana V et al. LIED-Liver: information, education and diagnosis. Methods Inf Med 1989; 31:284-297.

Consoli SM, Ben Said M, Jean J et al. Benefits of a computer-assisted education program for hypertensive patients compared with standard education tools. Patient Educ Couns 1995; 26:343-347.

Cooper G. Probabilistic and decision-theoretic systems in medicine. Artif Intell Med 1993; 5:289-292.

Cooper H, Hedges L, eds. Handbook of Research Synthesis. New York:Russell Sage Foundation, 1994.

Covell DG, Uman GC, Manning PR. Information needs in office practice: are they being met? Ann Int Med 1985; 103:596-599.

Cundick RM, Turner CW, Lincoln MJ et al. Iliad as a patient case simulator to teach medical problem solving. Proc Annu Symp Comput Appl Med Care 1989:13:902-906.

Cunningham AJ, Lockwood GA, Cunningham JA. A relationship between perceived self-efficacy and quality of life in cancer patients. Patient Educ Couns 1991; 17:71-78.

Davis DA, Thomson MA, Oxman AD et al. Evidence for the effectiveness of CME: a review of 50 randomized control trials. JAMA 1992; 268: 1111-1117.

Davis TC, Crouch MA, Wills G et al. The gap between patient reading comprehension and the readability of patient education materials. J Fam Pract 1990; 31:533-538.

Davis TC, Mayeaux EJ. Reading ability of parents compared with reading level of pediatric patient education materials. Pediatrics 1994; 93:460-468.

Dawes RM, Faust D, Meehl PE. Clinical versus actuarial judgment. Science 1989; 243:1668-1674.

de Dombal FT. Computer-aided decision support: in praise of level playing fields. Methods Inf Med 1994; 33:161-163.

de Dombal FT. Computer-aided diagnosis and decision-making in the acute abdomen. J R Coll Physicians 1975; 9:211-218.

de Dombal FT. Computer-assisted diagnosis in Europe. N Engl J Med 1994; 331:1238.

de Dombal FT. Ethical considerations concerning computers in medicine in the 1980s. J Med Ethics 1987; 13:179-184.

de Dombal FT. The diagnosis of acute abdominal pain with computer assistance: worldwide perspective. Ann Chir 1991; 45:273-277.

de Dombal FT, Leaper DJ, Horrocks JC et al. Human and computer-aided diagnosis of abdominal pain: further report with emphasis on performance of clinicians. Br Med J 1974; 1:376-380.

de Dombal FT, Leaper DJ, Staniland JR et al. Computer aided diagnosis of acute abdominal pain. Br Med J 1972; 2:9-13.

Demers RY, Altimore HM, Kleinman A et al. An exploration of the dimensions of illness behavior. J Fam Pract 1980; 11:1085-1092.

Diamond LW. A different view of ILIAD. MD Comput 1992; 9:76-77.

Dickersin K. Why register clinical trials?—Revisited. Control Clin Trials 1992; 13:170-177.

Dickersin K, Min YI, Meinert CL. Factors influencing publication of research results: follow-up of applications submitted to two institutional review boards. JAMA 1992; 267:374-378.

Doak CC, Doak LG, Root JH. Teaching Patients with Low Literacy Skills. Philadelphia: JB Lippincott, 1985.

Doyle HR, Parmanto B, Munro PW et al. Building clinical classifiers using incomplete observations—a neural network ensemble for hepatoma detection in patients with cirrhosis. Methods Inf Med 1995; 34:253-258.

East TD, Henderson S, Morris AH et al. Implementation issues and challenges for computerized clinical protocols for management of mechanical ventilation in ARDS patients. Proc Annu Symp Comput Appl Med Care 1989:583-587.

Eddy DM, Clanton CH. The art of diagnosis: solving the clinicopathological conference. N Engl J Med 1982; 306:1263-1269.

Elmore JG, Wells CK, Lee CH et al. Variability in radiologists' interpretation of mammograms. N Engl J Med 1994; 331:1493-1499.

Elstein AS, Friedman CP, Wolf FM et al. Effects of a decision support system on the diagnostic accuracy of users: a preliminary report. JAMIA 1996; 3:422-428.

Elstein AS, Shulman LS, Sprafka SA. Medical problem solving: an analysis of clinical reasoning. Cambridge, MA: Harvard University Press, 1978.

Elstein AS, Shulman LS, Sprafka SA. Medical problem solving: a ten-year retrospective. Eval Health Prof 1990; 13:5-36.

Emori TG, Culver DH, Horan TC et al. National Nosocomial Infections Surveillance System (NNIS): description of surveillance methodology. Am J Infect Control 1991; 19:19-35.

Ende J, Kazis L, Ash A et al. Measuring patients' desire for autonomy: decision making and information-seeking preferences among medical patients. J Gen Intern Med 1989; 4:23-30.

Engle EL. Attempts to use computers as diagnostic aids in medical decision making: a thirty-year experience. Perspect Biol Med 1992; 35:207-219.

Evans DA, Patel VL, eds. Cognitive Science in Medicine. Cambridge, MA: MIT Press, 1989.

Evans M, Pollock AV. A score system for evaluating random clinical trials of prophylaxis of abdominal surgical wound infection. Br J Surg 1985; 72:256-260.

Evans RS, Burke JP, Pestotnik SL et al. Prediction of hospital infections and selection of antibiotics using an automated hospital data base. Proc Annu Symp Comput Appl Med Care 1990:663-667.

Evans RS, Classen DC, Pestotnik SL et al. A decision support tool for antibiotic therapy. Proc Annu Symp Comput Appl Med Care 1995:651-655.

Evans RS, Larsen RA, Burke JP et al. Computer surveillance of hospital-acquired infections and antibiotic use. JAMA 1986; 256:1007-1011.

Evans RS, Pestotnik SL, Classen DC et al. Development of a computerized adverse drug event monitor. Proc Annu Symp Comput Appl Med Care 1991:23-27.

Ewigman BG, Crane JP, Frigoletto FD et al. RADIUS Study Group. N Eng J Med 1993; 329:821-827.

Feinstein AR. An analysis of diagnostic reasoning. I. The domains and disorders of clinical macrobiology. Yale J Biol Med 1973; 46:212-232.

Feinstein AR. An analysis of diagnostic reasoning. II. The strategy of intermediate decisions. Yale J Biol Med 1973; 46:264-283.

Feldman MJ, Barnett GO. An approach to evaluating the accuracy of DXplain. Comput Methods Programs Biomed 1991; 35:261-266.

Feldman SR, Quinlivan A. Illiteracy and the readability of patient education materials. A look at Health Watch. N C Med J 1994; 55:290-292.

Ferguson CH. Computers and the coming of the U.S. keiretsu. Harv Bus Rev 1990; 68:55-70.

Feste C, Anderson RM. Empowerment: from philosophy to practice. Patient Educ Couns 1995; 26:139-144.

First MB, Soffer LJ, Miller RA. QUICK (Quick Index to Caduceus Knowledge): Using the Internist-I/Caduceus knowledge base as an electronic textbook of medicine. Comput Biomed Res 1985; 18:137-165.

Fisher LA, Johnson TS, Porter D et al. Collection of clean voided urine specimen: a comparison among spoken, written, and computer-based instructions. Am J Public Health 1977; 67:640-644.

Flexner SB, Stein J, eds. The Random House College Dictionary, Revised Edition. New York: Random House, Inc., 1988:366.

Fontaine D, Le Beux P, Riou C et al. An intelligent Computer-Assisted Instruction system for clinical case teaching. Methods Inf Med 1994; 33:433-445.

Food and Drug Administration. FDA regulation of medical device software. (Document prepared for an FDA Software Policy Workshop, Sept. 3-4, 1996, National Institutes of Health, Bethesda, Md.). http://www.fda.gov//cdrh/ost/points.html.

Food and Drug Administration, Center for Devices and Radiological Health. Policy for the Regulation of Computer Products, draft, 13 November 1989. Rockville, Maryland:FDA, CDRH, 1989.

Fordham D, McPhee SJ, Bird JA et al. The cancer prevention reminder system. MD Comput 1990; 7:289-295.

Forrow L, Wartman SA, Brock DW. Science, ethics, and the making of clinical decisions. JAMA 1988; 259:3161-3167.

Forsythe DE, Buchanan BG, Osheroff JA et al. Expanding the concept of medical information: an observational study of physicians' information needs. Comput Biomed Res 1992; 25:181-200.

Franco A, King JD, Farr FL et al. An assessment of the radiological module of NEONATE as an aid in interpreting chest X-ray findings by nonradiologists. J Med Syst 1991; 15:277-286.

Freeman R. Intrapartum fetal monitoring—a disappointing story. N Engl J Med 1990; 322:624-626.

Friedman CP. Where's the science in medical informatics? JAMIA 1995; 2:65-67.

Friedman LM, Furberg CD, DeMets DL. Fundamentals of Clinical Trials. Littleton, MA: PSG Publishing Company, 1985.

Frolich MW, Miller PL, Morrow JS. PATHMASTER: modelling differential diagnosis as "dynamic competition" between systematic analysis and disease-directed deduction. Comput Biomed Res 1990; 23:499-513.

Frost RD, Gillenson ML. Integrated clinical decision support using an object-oriented database management system. Meth Inform Med 1993; 32:154-160.

Fu LS, Huff S, Bouhaddou O et al. Estimating frequency of disease findings from combined hospital databases: a UMLS project. Proc Annu Symp Comput Appl Med Care 1991:373-377.

Funnell MM, Donnelly MB, Anderson RM et al. Perceived effectiveness, cost, and availability of patient education methods and materials. Diabetes Educ 1992; 18:139-145.

Gabert HA, Stenchever MA. Continuous electronic monitoring of fetal heart rate during labor. Am J Obstet Gynecol 1973; 115:919-923.

Gardner RM. Computerized data management and decision making in critical care. Surg Clin N America 1985; 65:1041-1051.

Gardner RM, Cannon GH, Morris AH et al. Computerized blood gas interpretation and reporting system. IEEE Computer 1975; 8:39-45.

Gardner RM, Christiansen PD, Tate KE et al. Computerized continuous quality improvement methods used to optimize blood transfusions. Proc Annu Symp Comput Appl Med Care 1993:166-170.

Gardner RM, Golubjatnikov OK, Laub RM et al. Computer-critiqued blood ordering using the HELP system. Comput Biomed Res 1990; 23:514-528.

Gardner RM, Lundsgaarde HP. Evaluation of user acceptance of a clinical expert system. JAMIA 1994; 1:428-438.

GCP: Nordic and European Guidelines. Austin: Pharmaco Dynamics Research, 1990.

Gehlbach SH, Wilkinson WE, Hammond WE et al. Improving drug prescribing in a primary care practice. Med Care 1984; 22:193-201.

Geissbuhler A, Miller RA. A new approach to the implementation of direct care-provider order entry. Proc AMIA Fall Symp 1996:689-693.

Georgakis DC, Trace DA, Naeymi-Rad Fet al. A statistical evaluation of the diagnostic performance of MEDAS—the medical emergency decision assistance system. Proc Annu Symp Comput Appl Med Care 1990:815-819.

Ghosh A, Marks IM, Carr AC. Therapist contact and outcome of self-exposure treatment for phobias. Br J Psych 1988; 152:234-238.

Gigerenzer G, Hoffrage U. How to improve Bayesian reasoning without instruction: frequency formats. Psychol Rev 1995; 102:684-704.

Gill CJ. Medical expert systems: grappling with the issues of liability. High Tech Law J 1987; 1:483-520.

Gillispie MA, Ellis LBM. Computer-based patient education revisited. J Med Syst 1993; 17:119-125.

Giuse DA, Giuse NB, Bankowitz RA et al. Heuristic determination of quantitative data for knowledge acquisition in medicine. Comput Biomed Res 1991; 24:261-272.

Giuse DA, Giuse NB, Miller RA. A tool for the computer-assisted creation of QMR medical knowledge base disease profiles. Proc Annu Symp Comput Appl Med Care 1991:978-979.

Giuse DA, Giuse NB, Miller RA. Consistency enforcement in medical knowledge base construction. Artif Intell Med 1993; 5:245-252.

Giuse NB, Giuse DA, Miller RA et al. Evaluating consensus among physicians in medical knowledge base construction. Methods Inf Med 1993; 32:137-145.

Goldberg DE. Genetic Algorithms in Search, Optimization, and Machine Learning. Reading, MA: Addison-Wesley, 1989.

Goldstein MK, Clarke AE, Michelson D et al. Developing and testing a multimedia presentation of a health-state description. Med Decis Making 1994; 14:336-344.

Goodman KW. Bioethics and health informatics: an introduction. In: Goodman KW, ed. Ethics, Computing and Medicine: Informatics and the Transformation of Health Care. Cambridge and New York: Cambridge University Press, 1997:1-31.

Goodman KW. Outcomes, futility, and health policy research. In: Goodman KW, ed. Ethics, Computing and Medicine: Informatics and the Transformation of Health Care. Cambridge and New York: Cambridge University Press, 1997:116-138.

Goodman KW, ed. Ethics, Computing and Medicine: Informatics and the Transformation of Health Care. Cambridge and New York: Cambridge University Press, 1997.

Gorry A. Strategies for computer-aided diagnosis. Math Biosci 1968; 2:293-318.

Gorry GA, Barnett GO. Experience with a model of sequential diagnosis. Comput Biomed Res 1968; 1:490-507.

Gorry GA. Computer-assisted clinical decision making. Methods Inf Med 1973; 12:45.

Gough IR. Computer assisted diagnosis of the acute abdomen. Aust N Z J Surg 1993; 63:699-702.

Greenfield S, Kaplan S, Ware J Jr. Expanding patient involvement in care: effects on patient outcomes. Ann Intern Med 1985; 102:520-528.

Grzymala-Busse JW, Woolery LK. Improving prediction of preterm birth using a new classification scheme and rule induction. Proc Annu Symp Comput Appl Med Care 1994:730-734.

Guo D, Lincoln MJ, Haug PJ et al. Exploring a new best information algorithm for Iliad. Proc Annu Symp Comput Appl Med Care 1991:624-628.

Gustafson DH, Bosworth K, Hawkins RP et al. CHESS: a computer-based support system for providing information, referrals, decision support and social support to people facing medical and other health-related crises. Proc Annu Symp Comput Appl Med Care 1992:161-165.

Gustafson DH, Hawkins RP, Boberg EW et al. The impact of computer support on HIV infected individuals. Final report to the Agency for Health Care Policy and Research 1994.

Hafner AW, Filipowicz AB, Whitely WP. Computers in medicine: liability issues for physicians. Int J Clin Monit Comput 1989; 6:185-194.

Hammersley JR, Cooney K. Evaluating the utility of available differential diagnosis systems. Proc Annu Symp Comput Appl Med Care 1988:229-231.

Harris J. National Assessment of Consumer Health Information Demand and Delivery. in Summary Conference Report, Reference Point Foundation, Partnership for Networked Health Information for the Public, Rancho Mirage, CA. May 14-16, 1995. Washington, DC: Office of Disease Prevention and Health Promotion, DHHS, 1995:3-5.

Haynes RB, Walker CJ. Computer-aided quality assurance: a critical appraisal. Arch Intern Med 1987; 147:1297-1301.

Haug PJ, Clayton PD, Tocino I et al. Chest radiography: a tool for the audit of report quality. Radiol 1991; 180:271-276.

Haug PJ, Gardner RM, Tate KE et al. Decision support in medicine: examples from the HELP system. Comput Biomed Res 1994; 27:396-418.

Haug PJ, Pryor TA, Frederick PR. Integrating radiology and hospital information systems: the advantage of shared data. Proc Annu Symp Comput Appl Med Care 1992:187-191.

Haug PJ, Ranum DL, Frederick PR. Computerized extraction of coded findings from free-text radiology reports. Radiol 1990; 174:543-548.

Haug PJ, Rowe KG, Rich T et al. A comparison of computer-administered histories. Proc Annu Conf - Am Assoc Med Syst Inf Conf 1988:21-25.

Haug PJ, Warner HR, Clayton PD et al. A decision-driven system to collect the patient history. Comput Biomed Res 1987; 20:193-207.

Heathfield HA, Wyatt J. Philosophies for the design and development of clinical decision-support systems. Methods Inf Med 1993; 32:1-8.

Heckerling PS, Elstein AS, Terzian CG et al. The effect of incomplete knowledge on the diagnosis of a computer consultant system. Med Inf 1991;16:363-370.

Heckerman DE, Horvitz EJ, Nathwani BN. Toward normative expert systems: Part I. The Pathfinder project. Methods Inf Med 1992; 31:90-105.

Henderson S, East TD, Morris AH et al. Performance evaluation of computerized clinical protocols for management of arterial hypoxemia in ARDS patients. Proc Annu Symp Comput Appl Med Care 1989:588-592.

Herman PG, Gerson DE, Hessel SJ et al. Disagreements in chest roentgen interpretation. Chest 1975; 68:278-282.

Hershey CO, Porter DK, Breslau D et al. Influence of simple computerized feedback on prescription charges in an ambulatory clinic. Med Care 1986; 24:472-481.

Hickam DH, Shortliffe EH, Bischoff MB et al. The treatment advice of a computer-based cancer chemotherapy protocol advisor. Ann Intern Med 1985; 103:928-936.

Hippocrates. Prognosis. In Lloyd GER, ed. Hippocratic Writings, translated by Chadwick J, Mann WN. London: Penguin Books 1983,170-185.

Holman H, Lorig K. Patient education in the rheumatic diseases-pros and cons. Bull Rheum Dis 1987; 37:1-8.

Holman H, Mazonson P, Lorig K. Health education for self-management has significant early and sustained benefits in chronic arthritis. Trans Assoc Am Physicians 1989; 102:204-208.

Holt GA, Hallon JD, Hughes SE et al. OTC labels: can consumers read and understand them? Am Pharm 1990; 30:51-54.

Horvitz EJ, Heckerman DE. The inconsistent use of measures of certainty in artificial intelligence research. In: Uncertainty in Artificial Intelligence, Vol 1. Amsterdam; New York: Elsevier Science, 1986:137-151.

Horwitz RI. The experimental paradigm and observational studies of cause-effect relationships in clinical medicine. J Chronic Dis 1987; 40:91-99.

Hripcsak G, Clayton PD, Pryor TA et al. The Arden syntax for medical logic modules. Proc Annu Symp Comput Appl Med Care 1990:200-204.

Hubbard SM, Martin NB, Thurn AL. NCI's cancer information systems—bringing medical knowledge to clinicians. Oncology 1995; 9:302-309.

Hulse RK, Clark SJ, Jackson JC et al. Computerized medication monitoring system. Am J Hosp Pharm 1976; 33:1061-1064.

Hupp JA, Cimino JJ, Hoffer EF et al. DXplain — A computer-based diagnostic knowledge base. Medinfo 1986;5:117-121.

Hurst JW, Walker HK (eds). The Problem-Oriented System. New York, NY: Medcom Learning Systems, 1972.

Ingelfinger JA, Mosteller F, Thibodeau LA et al. Biostatistics in Clinical Medicine. New York: Macmillan, 1987.

Innis MD. Medisets. Computer-assisted diagnosis using a modified set theory. Proc Second Natl Health Conf, Health Informatics Conf, '94, Gold Coast Australia, 1994:286-291.

Israel BA, Sherman SJ. Social support, control and the stress process. In: Glanz K, Lewis FM, Rimer B, eds. Health Behavior and Health Education. San Francisco, CA:Jossey-Bass, 1990.

Isselbacher KJ, Braunwald E, Wilson JD, Martin JB, Fauci AS and Kasper DL, eds. Harrison's Principles of Internal Medicine, 13/e CD-ROM. New York: McGraw-Hill, 1995.

Jimison HB, Fagan LM, Shachter RD et al. Patient-specific explanation in models of chronic disease. Artif Intell Med 1992; 4:191-205.

Jimison HB, Henrion M. Hierarchical preference models for patients with chronic disease. Med Decis Making 1992; 7:351.

Jimison HB, Sher PP. Consumer health informatics: health information technology for consumers. J Am Soc Inf Sci 1995; 46:783-790.

Johnson DS, Ranzenberger J, Herbert RD et al. A computerized alert program for acutely ill patients. J Nurse Admin 1980; 10:26-35.

Johnson JA, Bootman HL. Drug-related morbidity and mortality: a cost of illness model. Arch Intern Med 1995; 155:1949-1956.

Johnston ME, Langton KB, Haynes RB et al. Effects of computer-based clinical decision support systems on clinician performance and patient outcome: a critical appraisal of research. Ann Intern Med 1994; 120:135-142.

Jubelirer SJ, Linton JC. Reading versus comprehension: implications for patient education and consent in an outpatient oncology clinic. J Cancer Educ 1994; 9:26-29.

Kahn CE, Roberts LM, Wang K et al. Preliminary investigation of a Bayesian network for mammographic diagnosis of breast cancer. Proc Annu Symp Comput Appl Med Care 1995:208-212.

Kahn G. Computer-based patient education: a progress report. MD Comput 1993; 10:93-99.

Kahn G. Computer-generated patient handouts. MD Comput 1993; 10:157-164.

Kahn MG, Fagan LM, Sheiner LB. Model-based interpretation of time-varying medical data. Proc Annu Symp Comput Appl Med Care 1989:28-32.

Kahn MG, Steib SA, Fraser VJ et al. An expert system for culture-based infection control surveillance. Proc Annu Symp Comput Appl Med Care 1993:171-175.

Kahneman D, Slovic P, Tversky A, eds. Judgment Under Uncertainty: Heuristics and Biases. Cambridge, UK: Cambridge University Press, 1982.

Kasper JF, Mulley AF Jr., Wennberg JE. Developing shared decision making programs to improve the quality of health care. Qual Rev Bull 1992; 18:183-190.

Kassirer JP, Gorry GA. Clinical problem-solving — a behavioral analysis. Ann Intern Med 1978; 89:245-255.

Kassirer JP. A report card on computer-assisted diagnosis—the grade: C. N Engl J Med 1994; 330:1824-1825.

Kassirer JP, Kopelman RI. Cognitive errors in diagnosis: instantiation, classification, and consequences. Am J Med 1989; 86:433-440.

Kessler DA, Pape SM, Sundwall DN. The federal regulation of medical devices. N Engl J Med 1987; 317:357-366.

Kieschnick T, Adler L, Jimison HB. 1996 Health Informatics Directory. Baltimore, MD: Williams and Wilkins, 1995.

Kohane IS. Temporal reasoning in medical expert systems. Medinfo1986; 5:170-174.

Kokol P, Mernik M, Zavrsnik J et al. Decision trees based on automatic learning and their use in cardiology. J Med Syst 1994; 18:201-206.

Kolodner JL, Leake DB. A tutorial introduction to case-based reasoning. In:Leake D, ed. Case-Based Reasoning: Experiences, Lessons and Future Directions. Cambridge, MA:AAAI Press/MIT Press, 1996:31-67.

Koran LM. The reliability of clinical methods, data, and judgments (second of two parts). N Engl J Med 1975; 293:695-701.

Korsch BM. What do patients and parents want to know? What do they need to know? Pediatrics 1984; 74:917-919.

Koton P. Reasoning about evidence in causal explanations. Proc Seventh Nat Conf Artif Intell 1988:256-261.

Kreps GL. Communication and health education: systems and applications. In: Brand R, Donohew L, eds. Communication and Health: Systems and Applications. Hillsdale, NJ: Lawrence Erlbaum Associates, 1990.

Kuperman GJ, Gardner RM, Pryor TA. HELP: A Dynamic Hospital Information System. New York: Springer-Verlag, 1991.

Kuperman GJ, Teich JM, Bates DW et al. Detecting alerts, notifying the physician, and offering action items: a comprehensive alerting system. Proc AMIA Fall Symp 1996:704-708.

Lange LL, Haak SW, Lincoln MJ et al. Use of Iliad to improve diagnostic performance of nurse practitioner students. J Nurs Educ 1997; 36:36-45.

Lau LM, Warner HR. Performance of a diagnostic system (Iliad) as a tool for quality assurance. Comput Biomed Res 1992; 25:314-323.

Laursen P. Event detection on patient monitoring data using causal probabilistic networks. Methods Inf Med 1994; 33:111-115.

Lee AS, Cutts JH, Sharp GC et al. AI/LEARN network. The use of computer-generated graphics to augment the educational utility of a knowledge-based diagnostic system (AI/RHEUM). J Med Syst 1987; 11:349-358.

Lepage EF, Gardner RM, Laub RM et al. Improving blood transfusion practice: role of a computerized hospital information system. Transfusion 1992; 32:253-259.

Leaper DJ, Horrocks JC, Staniland JR et al. Computer-assisted diagnosis of abdominal pain using "estimates" provided by clinicians. Br Med J 1972; 4:350-354.

Ledley RS, Lusted LB. Reasoning foundations of medical diagnosis. Science 1959; 130:9-21.

Levin M. Use of genetic algorithms to solve biomedical problems. MD Comput 1995; 12:193-199.

Li YC, Haug PJ, Warner HR. Automated transformation of probabilistic knowledge for a medical diagnostic system. Proc Annu Symp Comput Appl Med Care 1994:765-769.

Light RJ, Smith PV. Accumulating evidence: procedures for resolving contradictions among different research studies. Harvard Educational Review 1971; 41:420-471.

Lincoln MJ, Turner CW, Haug PJ et al. Iliad training enhances medical students' diagnostic skills. J Med Syst 1991; 15:93-109.

Lincoln MJ, Turner CW, Haug PJ et al. Iliad's role in the generalization of learning across a medical domain. Proc Annu Symp Comput Appl Med Care 1992:174-178.

Lindberg DA, Humphreys BL, McCray AT. The Unified Medical Language System. Methods Inf Med 1993; 32:281-291.

Lindberg DAB, Rowland LR, Buch CR Jr et al. CONSIDER: A computer program for medical instruction. Proc Ninth IBM Medical Symposium, 1968.

Lindberg DAB, Sharp GC, Kingsland LC et al. Computer based Rheumatology consultant. Medinfo1980:1311-1315.

Lipkin M, Engle Jr RL, Davis BJ et al. Digital computer as an aid to differential diagnosis. Arch Intern Med 1961; 108:124-140.

Lipkin M, Hardy JD. Differential diagnosis of hematological diseases aided by mechanical correlation of data. Science 1957; 125:551-552.

Lipkin M, Hardy JD. Mechanical correlation of data in differential diagnosis of hematological diseases. JAMA 1958; 166:113-123.

Llewellyn-Thomas HA, Thiel EC, Sem FWC et al. Presenting clinical trial information: a comparison of methods. Patient Educ Couns 1995; 25:97-107.

Lomas J; Enkin M; Anderson GM et al. Opinion leaders vs. audit and feedback to implement practice guidelines. JAMA 1991; 265:2202-2207.

Lomas MA, Anderson GM et al. Do practice guidelines guide practice? The effect of a consensus statement on the practice of physicians. N Engl J Med 1989; 321:1306-1311.

Long W. Medical diagnosis using a probabilistic causal network. Appl Artif Intell 1989; 3:367-383.

Lorig K, Chastain RL, Ung E et al. Development and evaluation of a scale to measure perceived self-efficacy in people with arthritis. Arthritis Rheum 1989; 32:37-44.

Lorig K, Seleznick M, Lubeck D et al. The beneficial outcomes of the arthritis self-management course are not adequately explained by behavior change. Arthritis Rheum 1989; 32:91-95.

Luger GF, Stubblefield WA. Artificial Intelligence and the Design of Expert Systems. Redwood City, CA: Benjamin/Cummings Publishing Company, Inc., 1989.

Lundsgaarde HP. Evaluating medical expert systems. Soc Sci Med 1987; 241:805-819.

Lyon HC, Healy JC, Bell JR et al. PlanAlyzer, an interactive computer-assisted program to teach clinical problem solving in diagnosing anemia and coronary heart disease. Acad Med 1992; 67:821-828.

Mahler HI, Kulik JA. Preferences for health care involvement, perceived control and surgical recovery: a prospective study. Soc Sci Med 1990; 31:743-751.

Maibach E, Flora J, Nass C. Changes in self-efficacy and health behavior in response to a minimal contact community health campaign. Health Communication 1991; 3:1-15.

Maiers JE. Fuzzy set theory and medicine: the first twenty years. Proc Annu Symp Comput Appl Med Care 1985:325-329.

Mann NH 3d, Brown MD. Artificial intelligence in the diagnosis of low back pain. Orthop Clin North Am 1991; 22:303-314.

Masys DR. Medical Informatics: glimpses of the promised land. Acad Med 1989; 64:13-14.

Massaro TA. Introducing physician order entry at a major academic medical center: I. Impact on organizational culture and behavior. Acad Med 1993; 68:20-25.

Mazoue JG. Diagnosis without doctors. J Med Philos 1990; 15:559-579.

McAdam WA, Brock BM, Armitage T et al. Twelve years experience of computer-aided diagnosis in a district general hospital. Ann R Coll Surg Engl 1990; 72:140-146.

McAlister NH, Covvey HD, Tong C et al. Randomized controlled trial of computer-assisted management of hypertension in primary care. Br Med J 1986; 293:670-674.

McDermott D, Doyle J. Non-monotonic logic-I. Artif Intell 1980; 13:41-72.

McDermott J. R1: A rule-based configurer of computer systems. Artif Intell 1982; 19:39-88.

McDonald CJ. Protocol-based computer reminders, the quality of care and the non-perfectibility of medicine. N Engl J Med 1976; 295:1351-1355.

McDonald CJ, Hui SL, Smith DM et al. Reminders to physicians from an introspective computer medical record: a two-year randomized trial. Ann Int Med 1984; 100:130-138.

McDonald D, Grant A, Sheridan-Pereira M et al. The Dublin randomized controlled trial of intrapartum fetal heart rate monitoring. Am J Obstet Gynecol 1985; 152:524-539.

McDowell I, Newell C, Rosser W. Comparison of three methods of recalling patients for influenza vaccination. Can Med Assoc J 1986; 135:991-997.

McPhee SJ, Bird JA, Jenkins CN et al. Promoting cancer screening: a randomized, controlled trial of three interventions. Arch Intern Med 1989; 149:1866-1872.

Melin AL, Bygren LO. Efficacy of the rehabilitation of elderly primary health care patients after short-stay hospital treatment. Med Care 1992; 30:1004-1015.

Middleton B, Shwe MA, Heckerman DE et al. Probabilistic diagnosis using a reformulation of the Internist-1/QMR knowledge base. II. Evaluation of diagnostic performance. Methods Inf Med 1991; 30:256-267.

Miller GA. The magical number seven, plus or minus two: some limits on our capacity for processing information. Psychol Rev 1956; 63:81-97.

Miller PL. A Critiquing Approach to Expert Computer Advice: ATTENDING. Boston: Pittman, 1984.

Miller PL. The evaluation of artificial intelligence systems in medicine. Comput Methods Programs Biomed 1986; 22:5-11.

Miller PL, Frawley SJ, Sayward FG et al. IMM/Serve: An Internet-Accessible Rule-Based Program for Childhood Immunization. Proc Annu Symp Comput Appl Med Care 1995:208-212.

Miller RA. Evaluating evaluations of medical diagnostic systems. JAMIA 1996; 3:429-431.

Miller RA. Internist-1/Caduceus: problems facing expert consultant programs. Methods Inf Med 1984; 23:9-14.

Miller RA. Legal issues related to medical decision-support systems. Int J Clin Monit Comput 1989; 6:75-80.

Miller RA. Medical diagnostic decision support systems—past, present, and future: a threaded bibliography and commentary. JAMIA 1994; 1:8-27.

Miller RA. Why the standard view is standard: people, not machines, understand patients' problems. J Med Philos 1990; 15:581-591.

Miller RA, Goodman KW. Ethical challenges in the use of decision-support software in clinical practice. In: Goodman KW, ed. Ethics, Computing and Medicine: Informatics and the Transformation of Health Care. Cambridge and New York: Cambridge University Press, 1997:102-115.

Miller RA, Giuse NB. Medical knowledge bases. Acad Med 1991; 66:15-17.

Miller RA, Masarie FE. Use of the Quick Medical Reference (QMR) program as a tool for medical education. Methods Inf Med 1989; 28:340-345.

Miller RA, Masarie FE Jr. The demise of the "Greek Oracle" model for medical diagnosis systems. Methods Inf Med 1990; 29:1-2.

Miller RA, Masarie FE Jr. The quick medical reference (QMR) relationships function: description and evaluation of a simple, efficient "multiple diagnoses" algorithm. Medinfo 1992:512-518.

Miller R, Masarie FE, Myers J. Quick Medical Reference (QMR) for diagnostic assistance. MD Comput 1986; 3:34-48.

Miller RA, McNeil MA, Challinor S et al. Status Report: The Internist-1 / Quick Medical Reference project. West J Med 1986; 145:816-822.

Miller RA, Pople HE Jr, Myers J. Internist-I, an experimental computer-based diagnostic consultant for general internal medicine. N Engl J Med 1982; 307:468-476.

Miller RA, Schaffner KF. The logic of problem-solving in clinical diagnosis: a course for second-year medical students. J Med Educ 1982; 57:63-65.

Miller RA, Schaffner KF, Meisel A. Ethical and legal issues related to the use of computer programs in clinical medicine. Ann Intern Med 1985; 102:529-536.

Minsky M. A framework for representing knowledge. In: Haugeland J, ed. Mind Design. Cambridge, MA: MIT Press, 1981:95-128.

Mitchell JA, Lee AS, TenBrinkT et al. AI/Learn: an interactive videodisk system for teaching medical concepts and reasoning. J Med Syst 1987; 11:421-429.

Moens HJ, van der Korst JK. Development and validation of a computer program using Bayes's theorem to support diagnosis of rheumatic disorders. Ann Rheum Dis 1992; 51:266-271.

Morgan PP. Illiteracy can have major impact on patients' understanding of health care information. Can Med Assoc J 1993; 148:1196-1197.

Morris AH, Wallace CJ, Menlove RL et al. A randomized clinical trial of pressure-controlled inverse ratio ventilation and extracorporeal CO_2 removal for adult respiratory distress syndrome. Am J Respir Crit Care Med 1994; 149:295-305.

Mortimer H. Computer-aided medicine: present and future issues of liability. Computer Law J 1989; 9:177-203.

Mullen PD, Laville EA, Biddle AK et al. Efficacy of psychoeducational interventions on pain, depression, and disability in people with arthritis: a meta-analysis. J Rheumatol 1987; 14 (Suppl 15):33-39.

Murphy GC, Friedman CP, Elstein AS. The influence of a decision support system on the differential diagnosis of medical practitioners at three levels of training. Proc AMIA Fall Symp Comput 1996:219-223.

Munsey RR. Trends and Events in FDA regulation of medical devices over the last fifty years. Food and Drug Law J 1995; 50:163-177.

Musen MA, van der Lei J. Knowledge engineering for clinical consultation programs: modeling the application area. Methods Inf Med 1989; 28:28-35.

Naranjo CA, Busto U, Sellers EM et al. A method for estimating the probability of adverse drug reactions. Clin Pharmacol Ther 1981; 30:239-245.

Nease RF Jr. Risk attitudes in gambles involving length of life: aspirations, variations, and ruminations. Med Decis Making 1994; 14:201-203.

Nelson SJ, Blois MS, Tuttle MS et al. Evaluating RECONSIDER: a computer program for diagnostic prompting. J Med Sys 1985; 9:379-388.

Newell A, Shaw JC, Simon HA. Elements of a theory of human problem solving. Psychol Rev 1958; 65:151-166.

Newell A, Simon HA. Human Problem Solving. Englewood Cliffs, NJ: Prentice Hall, 1972.

Nicolucci A, Grilli R, Alexian AA et al. Quality, evolution, and clinical implications of randomized controlled trials on the treatment of lung cancer. JAMA 1989; 262:2101-2107.

Nilasena DS, Lincoln MJ. A computer-generated reminder system improves physician compliance with diabetes preventive care guidelines. Proc Annu Symp Comput Appl Med Care 1995:640-645.

Norman GR, Tugwell P, Feightner JW et al. Knowledge and clinical problem-solving ability. Med Educ 1985; 19:344-356.

Olsen DM, Kane RL, Proctor PH. A controlled trial of multiphasic screening. N Eng J Med 1976; 294:925-930.

O'Leary A, Shoor S, Lorig K et al. A cognitive-behavioral treatment for rheumatoid arthritis. Health Psychol 1988; 7:527-544.

O'Leary A. Self-efficacy and health. Behav Res Ther 1985; 23:437-451.

O'Rourke K, Detsky AS. Meta-analysis in medical research: strong encouragement for higher quality in individual research efforts. J Clin Epidemiology 1989; 42:1021-1024.

O'Shea JS. Computer-assisted pediatric diagnosis. Am J Dis Child 1975; 129:199-202.

Ornstein SM, Garr DR, Jenkins RG et al. Computer-generated physician and patient reminders: tools to improve population adherence to selected preventive services. J Fam Pract 1991; 32:82-90.

Osheroff JA, Forsythe DE, Buchanan BG et al. Physicians' information needs: an analysis of questions posed during clinical teaching in internal medicine. Ann Intern Med 1991; 114:576-581.

Overhage JM, Tierney WM, McDonald CJ. Computer reminders to implement preventive care guidelines for hospitalized patients. Arch Intern Med 1996; 156:1551-1556.

Parker RC, Miller RA. Creation of realistic appearing simulated patient cases using the Internist-1/QMR knowledge base and interrelationship properties of manifestations. Methods Inf Med 1989; 28:346-351.

Paterson-Brown S, Vipond MN, Simms K et al. Clinical decision-making and laparoscopy versus computer prediction in the management of the acute abdomen. Br J Surg 1989; 76:1011-1013.

Patil R. Review of causal reasoning in medical diagnosis. Proc Annu Symp Comput Appl Med Care 1986:11-16.

Patil R, Szolovits P, Schwartz W. Causal understanding of patient illness and diagnosis. Proc Seventh Int Joint Conf Artif Intell 1981:893-899.

Patil S, Henry JW, Rubenfire M, et al. Neural network in the clinical diagnosis of pulmonary embolism. Chest 1993; 104:1685-1689.

Pauker SG, Gorry GA, Kassirer JP et al. Towards the simulation of clinical cognition. Taking a present illness by computer. Am J Med 1976; 60:981-996.

Pauker SG, Kassirer JP. Decision analysis. N Engl J Med 1987; 316:250-258.

Paul RH, Hon EH. Clinical fetal monitoring. V. Effect on perinatal outcome. Am J Obstet Gynecol 1974; 118:529-533.

Pearl J. Probabilistic Reasoning in Intelligent Systems: Networks of Plausible Inference. San Mateo, CA: Morgan-Kaufman, 1988.

Peck CC, Sheiner LB, Martin MM et al. Computer-assisted digoxin therapy. N Engl J Med 1973; 289:441-446.

Pestotnik SL, Classen DC, Evans RS et al. Implementing antibiotic practice guidelines through computer-assisted decision support: clinical and financial outcomes. Ann Int Med 1996; 124:884-890.

Peterson C, Stunkard AJ. Personal control and health promotion. Soc Sci Med 1989; 28:819-828.

Peterson MC, Holbrook JH, Von Hales D et al. Contributions of the history, physical examination, and laboratory investigation in making medical diagnoses. West J Med 1992; 156:163-166.

Petterson T. How readable are the hospital information leaflets available to elderly patients? Age Ageing 1994; 23:14-16.

Piantadosi S, Byar DP. A proposal for registering clinical trials. Control Clin Trials 1988; 9:82-84.

Pinciroli F, Combi C, Pozzi G. Object oriented DBMS techniques for time oriented medical records. Med Inf 1992; 17:231-241.

Pingree S, Hawkins RP, Gustafson DH et al. Will HIV-positive people use an interactive computer system for information and support? A study of CHESS in two communities. Proc Annu Symp Comput Appl Med Care 1993:22-26.

Pople HE Jr. Heuristic methods for imposing structure on ill-structured problems: the structuring of medical diagnostics. In Szolovits P, ed. Artificial Intelligence in Medicine. AAAS Symposium Series. Boulder, CO: Westview Press, 1982; 119-190.

Pople HE, Myers JD, Miller RA. DIALOG: A model of diagnostic logic for internal medicine. Proc Fourth Int Joint Conf Artif Intell1975:848-855

Porter D. Patient responses to computer counseling. Proc Annu Symp Comput Appl Med Care 1978:233-237.

Porter JF, Kingsland LCd, Lindberg DA et al. The AI/RHEUM knowledge-based computer consultant system in rheumatology. Performance in the diagnosis of 59 connective tissue disease patients from Japan. Arthritis Rheum 1988; 31:219-226.

Pozen MW, D'Agostino RB, Selker HP et al. A predictive instrument to improve coronary-care-unit admission practices in acute ischemic heart disease. N Engl J Med 1984; 310:1273-1278.

Pradhan M, Provan G, Henrion M. Experimental analysis of large belief networks for medical diagnosis. Proc Annu Symp Comput Appl Med Care 1994:775-779.

Privitera MD, Homan RW, Ludden TM et al. Clinical utility of a Bayesian dosing program for phenytoin. Ther Drug Monit 1989; 11:285-294.

Problem-Knowledge Coupler System. Burlington, VT: PKC Corporation, 1994.

Pryor TA, Clayton PD, Haug PJ et al. Design of a knowledge driven HIS. Proc Annu Symp Comput Appl Med Care 1987:60-63.

Public Law No. 94-295, 90 Stat. 539 (1976), codified at 21 U.S.C. Sections 360c et seq. (1982).

Public Law No. 75-717, 52 Stat. 1040 (1938), as amended 21 U.S.C. Sections 301 et seq. (1988).

Quick Medical Reference (QMR). Pittsburgh, PA: CAMDAT Corporation, 1992.

Quinlan JR. Induction in decision trees. Machine Learning 1986;1:81-106.

Raiffa H. Decision analysis. Reading, MA: Addison-Wesley Inc, 1970.

Raines CJ, McFarlane DV, Wall C. Audit procedures in the national breast screening study: mammography interpretation. J Can Assoc Radiol 1986; 37:256-260.

Reggia JA, Nau DS, Wang PY. Diagnostic expert systems based on a set covering model. Internat J Man-Machine Stud 1983; 19:437-460.

Reid JA, Kenny GNC. Evaluation of closed-loop control of arterial pressure after cardiopulmonary bypass. Br J Anaesth 1987; 59:247-255.

Reid JC, Klachko DM, Kardash CA et al. Why people don't learn from diabetes literature: influence of text and reader characteristics. Patient Educ Couns 1995; 25:31-38.

Reiter R. A logic for default reasoning. Artif Intell 1980; 13:81-132.

Rhea JT, Potsaid MS, DeLuca SA. Errors of interpretation as elicited by a quality audit of an emergency radiology facility. Radiol 1979; 132:277-280.

Robinson TN. Community health behavior change through computer network health promotion: preliminary findings from Stanford Health-Net. Comput Methods Programs Biomed 1989; 30:137-144.

Rodman JH, Jelliffe RW, Kolb E et al. Clinical studies with computer-assisted initial lidocaine therapy. Arch Intern Med 1984; 144:703-709.

Rosenbaum M, Leibel RL, Hirsch J. Obesity. N. Engl. J. Med 1997; 337:396-407.

Rubin DH, Leventhal JM, Sadock RT et al. Educational intervention by computer in childhood asthma: a randomized clinical trial testing the use of a new teaching intervention in childhood asthma. Pediatrics 1986; 77:1-10.

Russell S, Norvig P. Artificial Intelligence: A Modern Approach. Upper Saddle River: Prentice-Hall, 1995.

Rutledge GW, Andersen SK, Polaschek JX et al. A belief network model for interpretation of ICU data. Proc Annu Symp Comput Appl Med Care 1990:785-789.

Sacks HS, Berrier J, Reitman D et al. Meta-analyses of randomized controlled trials. N Engl J Med 1987; 316:450-455.

Safran C, Herrmann F, Rind D et al. Computer-based support of clinical decision making. MD Comput 1990; 9:319-322.

Schmidt HG, Norman GR, Boshuizen HPA. A cognitive perspective on medical expertise: theory and implications. Acad Med 1990; 65:611-621.

Schoolman HM. Obligations of the expert system builder: meeting the needs of the user. MD Comput 1991; 8:316-321.

Schoolman HM. The impact of electronic computers and other technologies on information resources for the physician. Bull N Y Acad Med 1985; 61:283-289.

Shafer G. A Mathematical Theory of Evidence. Princeton, NJ: Princeton University Press, 1976.

Shannon CE, Weaver W. The Mathematical Theory of Communication. Urbana: University of Illinois Press, 1949.

Sharhar Y, Musen M. A temporal-abstraction system for patient monitoring. Proc Annu Symp Comput Appl Med Care 1992:121-127.

Shiomi S, Kuroki T, Jomura H et al. Diagnosis of chronic liver disease from liver scintiscans by fuzzy reasoning. J Nuclear Med 1995; 36:593-598.

Shortliffe EH, Buchanan BG, Feigenbaum EA. Knowledge engineering for medical decision-making: a review of computer-based clinical decision aids. Proc IEEE 1979; 67:1207-1224.

Shortliffe EH, Buchanan BG. A model of inexact rea email: soning in medicine. Math Biosci 1975; 23:351-379.

Shortliffe EH. Computer-Based Medical Consultations: MYCIN. New York, NY: Elsevier Computer Science Library, Artificial Intelligence Series, 1976.

Shortliffe EH. The adolescence of AI in medicine: Will the field come of age in the '90s? Artif Intell Med 1993; 5:93-106.

Shortliffe EH, Perreault LE, eds. Medical Informatics. Reading, MA: Addison Wesley Publishing, 1990.

Shwe M, Sujansky W, Middleton B. Reuse of knowledge represented in the Arden syntax. Proc Annu Symp Comput Appl Med Care 1992:47-51.

Shy KK, Luthy DA, Bennett FC et al. Effects of electronic fetal heart-rate monitoring, as compared with periodic auscultation, on the neurologic development of premature infants. N Engl J Med 1990; 322:588-593.

Siegal JA, Parrino TA. Computerized diagnosis: implications for clinical education. Med Educ 1988; 22:47-54.

Simborg DW, Whiting-O'Keefe QE. Evaluation methodology for ambulatory care information systems. Med Care 1982; 20:255-265.

Simon HA. The structure of ill-structured problems. Artif Intell 1973; 4:181-201.

Sittig DF, Pace NL, Gardner RM et al. Implementation of a computerized patient advise system using the HELP clinical information system. Comput Biomed Res 1989; 22:474-487.

Skinner CS, Siegfried JC, Kegler MC et al. The potential of computers in patient education. Patient Educ Couns 1993; 22:27-34.

Skinner CS, Strecher VJ, Hospers H. Physicians' recommendations for mammography: do tailored messages make a difference? Am J Public Health 1994; 84:43-49.

Smith L. The coming health care shakeout. Fortune 1993; May 17:70-75.

Snapper JW. Responsibility for computer-based decisions in health care. In: Goodman KW, ed. Ethics, Computing and Medicine: Informatics and the Transformation of Health Care. Cambridge and New York: Cambridge University Press, 1997:43-56.

Sobel DS. Self-care in health: Information to empower people. In: Levy AH, Williams B. Proc Annu Conf - Am Assoc Med Syst Inf Conf 1987:12-125.

Soljak MA, Handford S. Early results from the Northland immunization register. N Z Med J 1987; 100:244-246.

Sonnenberg FA, Hagerty CG, Kulikowski CA. An architecture for knowledge-based construction of decision models. Med Decis Making 1994; 14:27-39.

Sorace JM, Berman JJ, Carnahan GE et al. PRELOG: precedence logic inference software for blood donor deferral. Proc Annu Symp Comput Appl Med Care 1991:976-977.

Sox HC, Blatt MA, Higgins MC et al. Medical Decision Making. Boston: Butterworth-Heinemann, 1988.

Spilker B. Guide to Clinical Trials. New York: Raven, 1991.

Stamper R, Todd BS, Macpherson P. Case-based explanation for medical diagnostic programs, with an example from gynaecology. Methods Inf Med 1994; 33:205-213.

Starmer CF, Lee KL, Harell FE et al. On the complexity of investigating chronic illness. Biometrics 1980; 36:333-335.

Stead WW et al. Designing medical informatics research and library-resource projects to increase what is learned. JAMIA 1994; 1:28-34.

Su MC. Use of neural networks as medical diagnosis expert systems. Comput Biol Med 1994; 24:419-429.

Suryanarayanan S, Reddy NP, Canilang EP. A fuzzy logic diagnosis system for classification of pharyngeal dysphagia. Int J Biomed Comput 1995; 38:207-215.

Sutton GC. How accurate is computer-aided diagnosis? Lancet 1989; 2:905-908.

Swender PT, Tunnessen WW Jr, Oski FA. Computer-assisted diagnosis. Am J Dis Child 1974; 127:859-861.

Szolovits P, Pauker SG. Categorical and probabilistic reasoning in medical diagnosis. Artif Intell 1978; 11:114-144.

Tape TG, Campbell JR. Computerized medical records and preventive health care: success depends on many factors. Am J Med 1993; 94:619-625.

Tate KE, Gardner RM. Computers, quality and the clinical laboratory: a look at critical value reporting. Proc Annu Symp Comput Appl Med Care 1993:193-197.

Tate KE, Gardner RM, Scherting K. Nurses, pagers, and patient-specific criteria: three keys to improved critical value reporting. Proc Annu Symp Comput Appl Med Care 1995:164-168.

Tate KE, Gardner RM, Weaver LK. A computer laboratory alerting system. MD Comput 1990; 7:296-301.

Teach RL, Shortliffe EH. An analysis of physician attitudes regarding computer-based clinical consultation systems. Comput Biomed Res 1981; 14:542-558.

Teich JM, Geisler MA, Cimermann DE et al. Design considerations in the BWH ambulatory medical record: features for maximum acceptance by clinicians. Proc Annu Symp Comput Appl Med Care 1990:735-739.

Thompson SC, Pitts JS, Schwankovsky L. Preferences for involvement in medical decision-making: situational and demographic influences. Patient Educ Couns 1993; 22:133-140.

Tierney WM, Hui SL, McDonald CJ. Delayed feedback of physician performance versus immediate reminders to perform preventive care. Med Care 1986; 24:659-666.

Tierney WM, Miller ME, McDonald CJ. The effect on test ordering of informing physicians of the charges for outpatient diagnostic tests. N Engl J Med 1990; 322:1499-1504.

Tierney WM, Overhage JM, McDonald CJ. Computerizing guidelines: factors for success. Proc AMIA Fall Symp 1996:459-462.

Tierney WM, Overhage JM, McDonald CJ. Toward electronic records that improve care. Ann Intern Med 1995; 122:725-726.

Tu SW, Eriksson H, Gennari JH et al. Ontology-based configuration of problem-solving methods and generation of knowledge-acquisition tools: application of PROTEGE-II to protocol-based decision support. Artif Intell Med 1995; 7:257-289.

Turley TM. Expert software systems: the legal implications. Computer Law J 1988; 8:455-477.

Turner CW, Williamson JW, Lincoln MJ et al. The effects of Iliad on medical student problem solving. Proc Annu Symp Comput Appl Med Care 1990:478-482.

Tversky A, Kahneman D. Judgment under uncertainty: heuristics and biases. Science 1974; 188:1124-1131.

Tyson JE, Furzan JA, Resich JS et al. An evaluation of the quality of therapeutic studies in perinatal medicine. J Pediatr 1983; 102:10-13.

Van Schoonhoven P, Berkmann EM, Lehman R, Fromberg R, eds. Medical Staff Monitoring Functions-Blood Usage Review. Chicago: Joint Commission on Accreditation of Hospitals, 1987.

Vinicor F, Cohen SJ, Mazzuca SA et al. DIABEDS: a randomized trial of the effects of physician and/or patient education on diabetes patient outcomes. J Chronic Dis 1987; 40:345-356.

Voytovich AE, Rippey RM, Suffredini A. Premature conclusions in diagnostic reasoning. J Med Educ 1985; 60:302-307.

Waitzkin H. Doctor-patient communication: clinical implications of social scientific research. JAMA 1984; 252:2441-2446.

Warner HR. Computer-Assisted Medical Decision Making. New York: Academic Press, 1979.

Warner HR Jr. Iliad: moving medical decision-making into new frontiers. Methods Inf Med 1989; 28:370-372.

Warner HR, Haug P, Bouhaddou O et al. ILIAD as an expert consultant to teach differential diagnosis. Proc Annu Symp Comput Appl Med Care 1987:371-376.

Warner HR, Rutherford BD, Houtchens B. A sequential Bayesian approach to history taking and diagnosis. Comput Biomed Res 1972; 5:256-262.

Warner HR, Toronto AF, Veasey LG et al. Mathematical approach to medical diagnosis. JAMA 1961; 177:75-81.

Waxman HS and Worley WE. Computer-assisted diagnosis. Ann Intern Med 1990; 113:561.

Waxman HS, Worley WE. Computer-assisted adult medical diagnosis: subject review and evaluation of a new microcomputer-based system. Medicine 1990; 69:125-136.

Weed LL. Knowledge Coupling: New Premises and New Tools for Medical Care and Education. New York, NY:Springer-Verlag, 1991.

Weed LL. Medical records that guide and teach. N Engl J Med 1968; 278:593-600 and 652-657.

Weed LL. Physicians of the future. N Engl J Med 1981; 304:903-907.

Weed LL. Problem-knowledge couplers: Philosophy, use and interpretation. PKC Corporation 1982:2-22.

Weed LL. Reengineering medicine: questions and answers. Federation Bull 1995; 82(1):24-36.

Weiss S, Kulikowski CA, Safir A. Glaucoma consultation by computer. Comput Biol Med 1978; 8:24-40.

Weiss S, Kulikowski CA. EXPERT: a system for developing consultation models. Proc Sixth Int Joint Conf Artif Intell 1979.

Weiss SM, Kulikowski CA, Amarel S et al. A model-based method for computer-aided medical decision making. Artif Intell 1978; 11:145-172.

Welford CR. A comprehensive computerized patient record with automated linkage to QMR. Proc Annu Symp Comput Appl Med Care 1994:814-818.

Wetstone SL, Sheehan TJ, Votaw RG et al. Evaluation of a computer based education lesson for patients with rheumatoid arthritis. J Rheumatol 1985; 12:907-912.

Wexler JR, Swender PT, Tunnessen WW Jr et al. Impact of a system of computer-assisted diagnosis. Initial evaluation of the hospitalized patient. Am J Dis Child 1975; 129:203-205.

Wheeler LA, Brecher G, Sheiner LB. Clinical laboratory use in the evaluation of anemia. JAMA 1977; 238:2709-2714.

Willems JL, Abreu-Lima C, Arnaud P et al. The diagnostic performance of computer programs for the interpretation of electrocardiograms. N Engl J Med 1991; 325:1767-1773.

Williams LS. Microchips versus stethoscopes: Calgary hospital, MDs face off over controversial computer system. Can Med Assoc J 1992; 147: 1534-1547.

Williamson JW, German PS, Weiss R et al. Health science information management and continuing education of physicians - a survey of U.S. primary care practitioners and their opinion leaders. Ann Intern Med 1989; 110:151-160.

Williamson JW, Goldschmit PG, Colton T. The quality of medical literature: an analysis of validation assessments. In: Bailar, JC 3rd, Mosteller, F, eds. Medical Uses of Statistics, Walton, MA: NEJM Books, 1986:370-391.

Wones RG. Failure of low-cost audits with feedback to reduce laboratory test utilization. Med Care 1987; 25:78-82.

Wu Y, Giger ML, Doi K et al. Artificial neural networks in mammography: application to decision making in the diagnosis of breast cancer. Radiology 1993; 187:81-87.

Wyatt J, Spiegelhalter D. Field trials of medical decision-aids: potential problems and solutions. Proc Annu Symp Comput Appl Med Care 1991:3-7.

Yerushalmy J. Reliability of chest radiology in the diagnosis of pulmonary lesions. Am J Surg 1955; 89:231-240.

Yolton RL. Computer-based diagnostic systems. N Engl J Med 1994; 331:1023.

Young FE. Validation of medical software: present policy of the Food and Drug Administration. Ann Intern Med 1987; 106:628-629.

Yu VL, Fagan LM, Wraith SM et al. Antimicrobial selection by computer: a blinded evaluation by infectious disease experts. JAMA 1979; 242: 1279-1282.

Yu H, Haug PJ, Lincoln MJ, Turner C, Warner HR. Clustered knowledge representation: Increasing the reliability of computerized expert systems. Proc Annu Symp Comput Appl Med Care 1988:126-130.

Yu VL. Conceptual obstacles in computerized medical diagnosis. J Med Phil 1983; 8:67-75.

Zadeh LA. Fuzzy logic, neural networks, and soft computing. Comm of ACM 1994; 37:77-84.

Ziegler DK, Hurwitz A, Hassanein RS et al. Migraine prophylaxis: a comparison of Propranolol and Amitriptyline. Arch Neurol 1987; 44:486-489.

Zimmerman HJ. Fuzzy Set Theory and Its Applications. 2nd ed. Amsterdam: Kluwer-Nijhoff, 1990.

INDEX

A

Abdominal pain system. *See* Leeds abdominal pain system.
ABEL, 176, 182-183
Acute abdominal pain system. *See* Leeds abdominal pain system.
AI/Learn, 127
AI/Rheum, 16, 55, 127
AMA Family Medical Guide, 149-150, 153, 158-160
Antibiotic assistant, 93-94, 107

B

Bayes' theorem, 8, 11, 13-15, 18, 45-48, 53-55, 57, 95-96, 98, 109-110, 121, 123, 132, 154, 173, 179, 181, 183-185
Bayesian belief network, 15, 18, 110, 173
conditional independence, 181, 183-184
Boolean algebra, 11, 14, 39

C

CADUCEUS, 113-115, 182
CANCERNET, 146
CASNET, 20, 169, 176, 181-183
CHF Advisor, 176, 182
Common sense knowledge. *See* Knowledge representation, default knowledge.
CONSIDER, 16
Consumers. *See* patient decision support system.

D

DeDombal system. *See* Leeds abdominal pain system.
Diagnosis, 3-6, 8-11, 13, 15-18, 20, 23-25, 28-29, 42, 45, 47, 49-50, 52-53, 55-56, 58, 61-68, 77, 89, 90-91, 98, 107, 110-112, 114, 116-117, 122-124, 126-129, 149, 152, 155-156, 158, 160, 170, 173, 177, 180-182, 184, 189, 191-192, 194, 200, 208, 210, 217-218, 220-222, 224, 227-228, 230-231

correct diagnosis, 11, 63-66, 117, 124, 181, 184, 194
decision making, 9, 38, 64, 93, 95, 105-106, 139, 141-143, 153, 181, 184, 194, 200-201, 211-212, 224-225
definition, 4, 6, 13, 16, 20, 27, 63, 202
diagnostic error, 111-112, 119-120, 133, 221
error avoidance, 220-221, 231
diagnostician, 3, 5-6, 9, 11, 13, 66-67
diagnostic process, 5-7, 9, 22, 63, 88-90, 92-95, 111, 182, 194
differential diagnosis, 11, 24, 50, 58, 110, 116, 122-124, 128, 191
gold standard, 15, 20, 25-26, 28, 97, 115, 125-127, 151, 209
hypotheses, 5, 9-12, 16, 23, 62, 69, 111-113, 116-120, 128, 181-182, 191, 203, 205-206
problem solving, 9, 111-112, 128
ill-structured problem, 10, 12
DXplain, 17, 28, 49, 56, 62, 113, 121-122, 129, 170

E

Education
medical student, 68, 116, 118, 120-121
teaching, 108, 110, 112, 115-119, 123, 125-127, 130, 132, 143
nurse practitioner, 119-121
patient. *See* Health Education
physician assistant, 121
problem-based learning, 106, 108
Ethics, 217-225
care standards, 219
community standard, 220
reasonable person, 220
Evaluation of decision support system, 61-70, 220
boundaries, 18, 23, 25
formative evaluation, 125
limitations, 18, 22, 23, 25, 50, 51, 58, 65, 182, 188, 194, 205, 218
needs assessment, 18, 162

performance, 8, 15, 17-18, 20, 24-26, 30, 62-63, 65-67, 69-70, 105, 110, 118, 120, 124-125, 127, 129-130, 170, 178, 186, 188-200, 202-203
Performance Standards, 66
randomized controlled trial, 69, 202, 205-207, 209, 211-212
sensitivity, 65, 92, 109-110, 117
specificity, 64-66, 109-110, 133
validity, 20, 112, 130-131, 133, 179

F

Food and Drug Administration (FDA), 28, 228, 230-231
devices, 28, 228-230
accessories, 228-229
components, 24, 50-51, 57, 211, 223, 228-229
educational and bibliographic software, 228
stand-alone software, 229
Food, Drug and Cosmetic Act, 228
Fuzzy logic. *See* Set theory, fuzzy set theory.

G

Germwatcher, 42

H

Health education, 139, 142, 161-162
empowerment, 140-141
patient preferences, 141-142
self-efficacy, 140-141
shared decision making, 143, 153, 224-225
Health Evaluation Through Logical Processes (HELP) system, 78-81, 85, 88-89, 90, 93, 95, 115, 204
HEME, 15, 16
Hepaxpert, 54
Home Medical Advisor Pro, 149-150, 156-158

I

Iliad, 17, 28, 48, 54, 62, 108-110, 113, 115-119, 121-122, 126, 128-133, 153-155, 170, 177
IMM/Serve, 54

Inference engine, 53-55, 107-108, 110, 115, 121, 128, 153, 155
reasoning, 9-17, 20, 35, 41-42, 48-50, 52-54, 56, 58, 65, 111, 114, 171, 173, 176, 178-179, 181-187, 191, 194
algorithm, 6, 12-13, 18, 108-109, 114, 125, 128, 153, 156, 186, 188-189, 191, 211
case-based reasoning, 186
causal reasoning, 10, 12, 181, 182
certainty factor, 48, 49, 180, 181
decision theory, 132, 184
decision trees, 132, 174, 188
heuristic, 10-11, 15-18, 48, 58, 109-110
hypothetico-deductive method, 10
informal logic, 48
pattern recognition, 9-10, 13, 94, 187
predicate logic, 40-41, 54
propositional logic, 172, 179-180
Internet. *See* World Wide Web.
Internist-1, 17-18, 113-115

K

Knowledge base, 16, 19-21, 23, 25-26, 28-30, 48-50, 55-56, 58, 62-63, 65, 67, 70, 86, 94, 106-111, 114-116, 121-128, 132, 153, 155, 170-173, 175, 177-183, 185-187, 191-192, 230
construction, 19-21, 30
data representation, 174
database management system, 118, 172, 174-175
object-oriented database, 175
relational database, 174
structured query language, 175
knowledge acquisition bottleneck, 187
knowledge acquisition tool, 110
knowledge engineering, 109-110, 115, 123, 127, 187, 208, 211
knowledge representation, 171-174, 176-177, 187, 193-194
causal modeling, 178, 182
clusters, 109
criteria tables, 16
default knowledge, 177
disease profile, 109-110, 114-115, 123, 127
frames, 54-55, 79, 96, 109, 126, 128, 143, 174, 211

procedural knowledge, 173
  temporal factors, 52
maintenance, 19-21, 50, 55
Knowledge-based system, 56, 62, 186
  rule-based system, 17, 91, 110, 173,
    180-181
    backward chaining, 17, 110, 124
    forward chaining, 17, 124
    IF-THEN rules, 12, 127
    production rules, 12, 54, 211

L

LDS Hospital. *See* HELP system.
Leeds abdominal pain system, 169-170,
  181
Legal issues
  liability, 226-227, 230
  negligence, 226-227
  regulation, 28-29, 226, 228, 230-231
  software quality audit, 28
Liver: Information, Education and
  Diagnosis (LIED), 128-129

M

Machine learning, 58, 187-188, 194
Mammonet, 54
Medical HouseCall, 149-150, 153, 156
Medical Matrix, 145
Meditel, 16, 28, 62, 129
MEDLINE, 35, 37, 39-40, 44, 58, 106,
  115, 131, 208
MYCIN, 17, 21, 42-43, 48-49, 54, 129,
  169, 173, 177-178, 180-181

N

NEONATE, 126-127
Non-knowledge-based system, 56, 58
  genetic algorithm, 57-58, 191
  neural network, 18, 56-58, 110, 174,
    187, 189-191

P

Pathfinder, 170, 178, 184
PATHMASTER, 122-123
Patient decision support system, 142
  design guidelines, 142
  drug information, 151-152
  Emergency First Aid, 152

home references, 144, 149
Library Reference Database, 150
patient access, 159
PDQ, 146
Pediatric HouseCall, 149-150, 153-156
PIP (Present Illness Program), 16
PKC (Problem Knowledge Coupler), 192
PlanAlyzer, 124-126
Probability, 8, 35-36, 39, 43-49, 54, 56,
  58, 93, 95, 98, 110, 116-120, 123, 126,
  180-181, 183-185
  conditional probability, 44-45, 58, 183
  posterior probability, 110, 117-120,
    123
  prior probability, 185

Q

QMR (Quick Medical Reference), 6, 17,
  28-29, 49, 62, 69, 108-110, 113-116,
  122, 128-129, 170, 177, 183, 187
  disease profiles, 110, 114-115, 127
  evoking strength, 49, 109, 110, 114
  findings, 6-7, 69, 114-115
  frequency, 49, 109-110, 114

R

RECONSIDER, 16
RESUME, 176

S

Set theory, 14, 18, 36, 39, 58, 185
  Boolean algebra, 11, 14, 39
  cardinality, 36
  element, 36-39, 52, 78, 80, 185
  fuzzy set theory, 18, 39
  intersection, 37, 38, 44
  locality, 179-181
  set covering, 18, 38
  subset, 15, 36, 38, 86, 92, 188
  union, 37, 38
System structure/function
  automated data entry, 67, 70
  browsing mode, 111, 115-116
  controlled vocabulary, 50, 52, 64
  critique function
    critiquing system, 83, 86
  electronic textbook, 23, 69, 111,
    113-114

Greek Oracle, 7, 17
input, 6-7, 13, 18-19, 22, 24, 26, 35,
    49-53, 56-58, 62, 68, 149, 154,
    177, 188-190, 192
output, 7-8, 14, 18, 24, 30, 49-50, 53,
    56, 58, 68, 80, 94, 171, 188-190,
    192, 223, 224
simulation mode, 111, 113-114, 116,
    118
standard view, 218-219
suggestion system, 86

T

The Family Doctor, 149
TOPAZ, 177

U

University of Rennes Computer-Assisted
    Instruction (CAI), 123, 124

Users
    appropriate use, 93, 219, 221-223, 231
    attitudes, 141, 193, 203-204
    critical mass, 22
    human-computer interaction, 171
    information needs, 5, 18, 23, 147-148
    integration, 5, 70, 170-171, 193
    user interface, 19, 21-22, 50, 62, 126,
        128
    user satisfaction, 203

W

World Wide Web, 144-145, 152, 227, 231

Health Informatics

(formerly Computers in Health Care)

(continued from page ii)

Trauma Informatics
K.I. Maull and J.S. Augenstein

Knowledge Coupling
New Premises and New Tools for Medical Care and Education
L.L. Weed